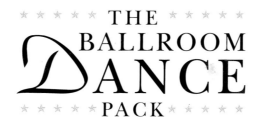

THE
BALLROOM
DANCE
PACK

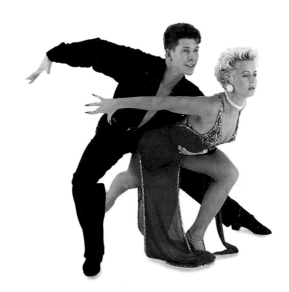

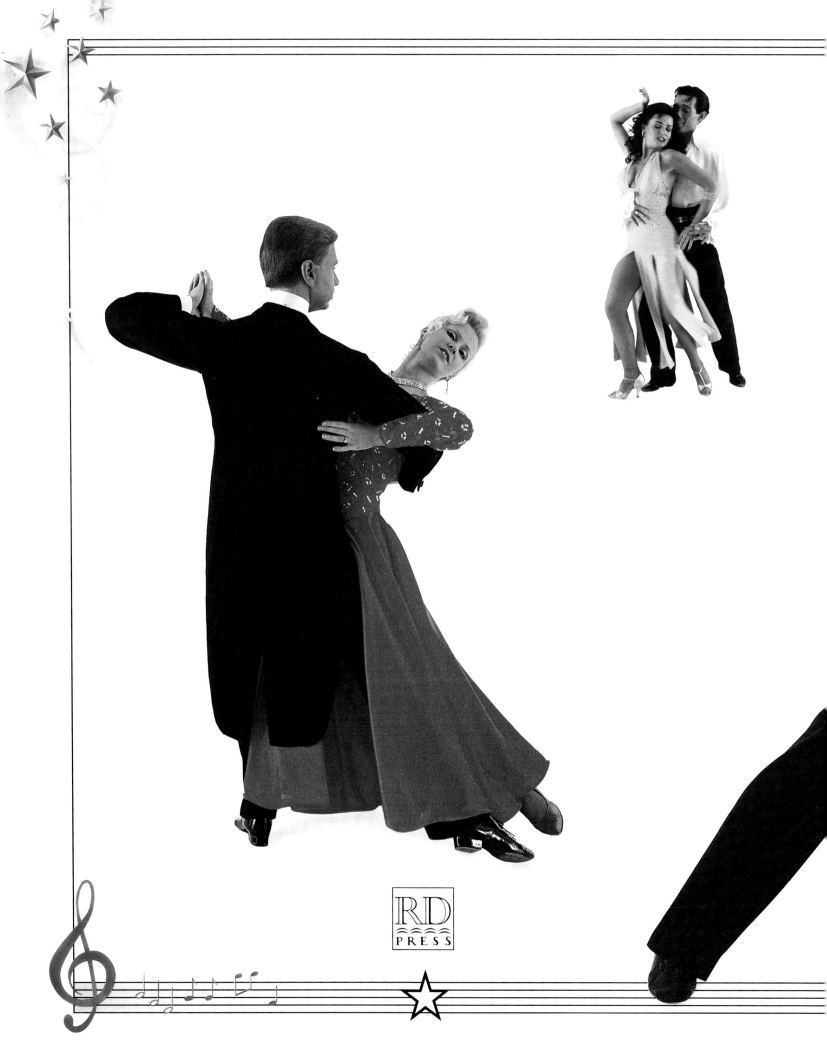

RD
PRESS

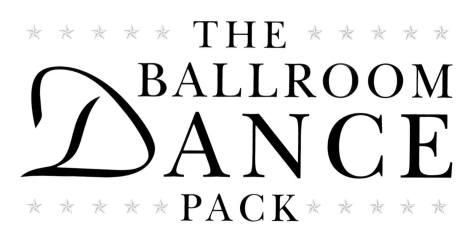

THE
BALLROOM
DANCE
PACK

WALTER LAIRD

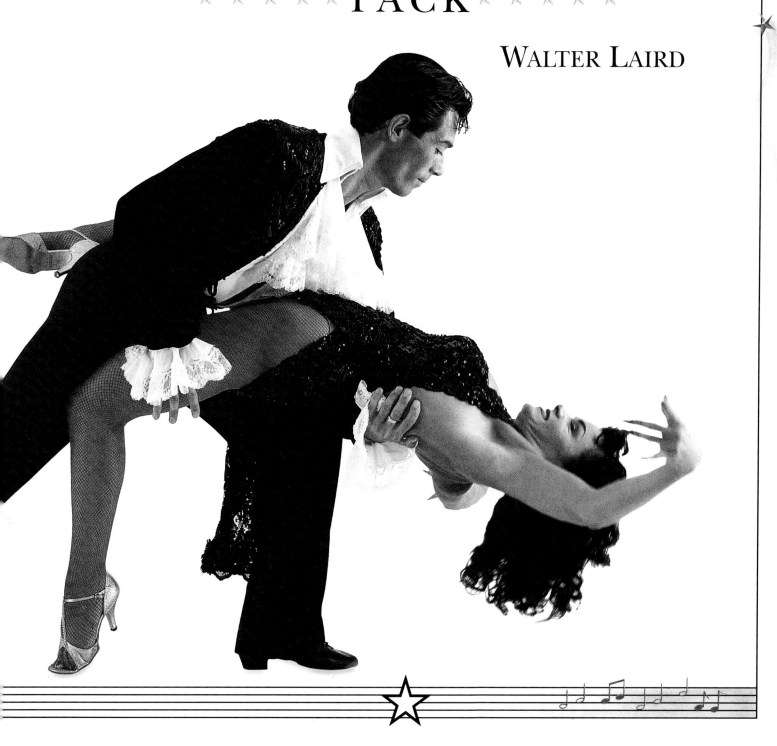

It takes two to Tango and it took two to write this dance book.
Thank you JULIE for all your help. W. L.

A DORLING KINDERSLEY BOOK

First published in Australia in 1994 by RD Press
a registered business name of
Reader's Digest (Australia) Pty Limited
26-32 Waterloo Street, Surry Hills, NSW 2010

Created and produced by
CARROLL & BROWN LIMITED
5 Lonsdale Road
London NW6 6RA

ISBN 0 86438 682 6

Reproduced by Colourscan, Singapore
Printed and bound by Tien Wah Press, Singapore

CONTENTS

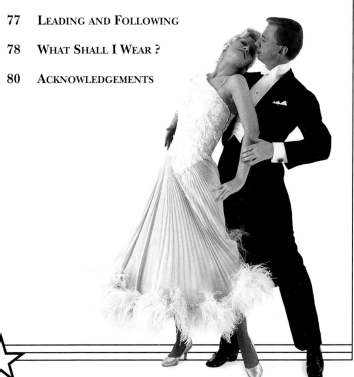

How To Use The Pack

THE BALLROOM DANCE PACK was created to help you master six of the world's most popular social dances. It contains everything you need to know to be able to take to any dance floor with ease and confidence. And once you are there, I guarantee that you will wonder why it took you so long to take the plunge. Enjoy!

THE BOOK

On the following pages, you will be introduced to both the Modern and Latin styles of ballroom dancing. Three dances from each of these styles are covered. Two championship couples, one a specialist in the Modern style and the other a specialist in the Latin style, have been photographed to show every foot, body, and arm position necessary to dance each figure.

DANCE INSTRUCTIONS
These employ a number of abbreviations. If only one instruction is given, this is directed to the man; his partner assumes the normal opposite position.

M ~
RF forward

W ~ LF back

The book also contains the following:

General background information
To introduce each dance, I've given some of its history, its country of origin and later evolution, and useful

advice on how to achieve a good quality performance. This is illustrated by action shots of our dancers in their competition clothes.

A Solo Exercise for each dance
You should practise these to perfect the basic actions required; each is shown in photographs, and charted out on The Dance Cards.

A selection of the most important basic figures for each dance
These are photographed step by step, and annotated with the correct timing and foot positions. **Learn each of these figures in the order they are given**; this is the natural order in which to dance them.

Figures, Amalgamations, and Routines; Leading and Following, and What Shall I Wear?
Some essential information that will add to your dancing pleasure can be found in The Appendix.

THE "LANGUAGE" OF BALLROOM DANCING

In common with many other activities, special words, phrases, and abbreviations are used to describe the nuts and bolts of ballroom dancing. While many of the more abstruse terms have been avoided, a few abbreviations are used throughout for reasons of space and clarity. These are listed below. For a fuller explanation of these and other terms used in the book, turn to THE GLOSSARY on page 75.

M	Man	CPP	Counter promenade position
W	Woman	OPEN CPP	Open counter promenade position
RF	Right foot		
LF	Left foot	OPEN PP	Open promenade position
LOD	Line of dance	PP	Promenade position

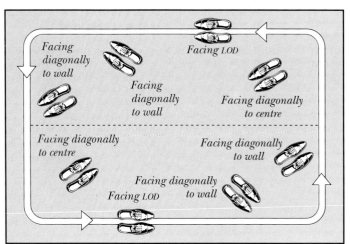

Facing diagonally to wall

Facing LOD

Facing diagonally to wall

Facing diagonally to centre

Facing diagonally to centre

Facing diagonally to wall

Facing LOD

Facing diagonally to wall

Unless stated otherwise, all instructions in the book, and in ballroom dance instructions in general, are directed at the man. The woman, therefore, must assume that the instruction requires her to dance the normal opposite to the man. For example, the normal opposite to "RF forward (Man)" is "LF back (Woman)". This methodology is adopted because ballroom dancing is a free-style dance form during which the man leads the woman, and the woman follows her partner's lead.

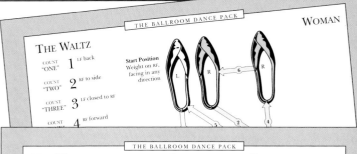

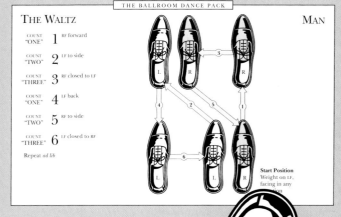

THE DANCE CARDS

As a reference guide to the SOLO EXERCISES, the man's and woman's steps for each have been printed on separate cards that can be held in the hand when practising.

THE DANCE CARDS

THE DANCING SHOES

Foot templates, in the shape of a man's and woman's pair of shoes, are included; these should be traced or photocopied as required and then cut out. Use them in conjunction with the foot patterns given for the SOLO EXERCISES; place in position as guides for your feet.

THE COMPACT DISC

Specially recorded dance music will help you perfect your dancing. There are two tracks of music for each of the dances included in the book. One track for each dance has been recorded at a slow tempo – use these tracks when you are learning the figures; the second track is normal dance tempo. Once you've mastered all the Modern or Latin dances, you can segue from dance to dance using the last two tracks.

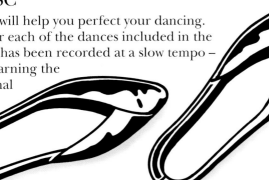

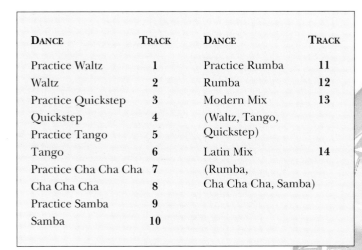

THE DANCING SHOES

THE COMPACT DISC

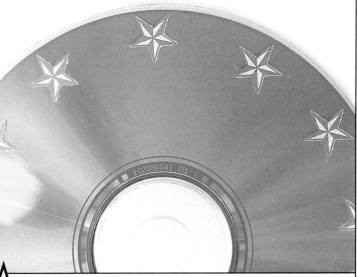

DANCE	TRACK	DANCE	TRACK
Practice Waltz	1	Practice Rumba	11
Waltz	2	Rumba	12
Practice Quickstep	3	Modern Mix	13
Quickstep	4	(Waltz, Tango,	
Practice Tango	5	Quickstep)	
Tango	6	Latin Mix	14
Practice Cha Cha Cha	7	(Rumba,	
Cha Cha Cha	8	Cha Cha Cha, Samba)	
Practice Samba	9		
Samba	10		

Ballroom Dancing ~ An Introduction

To dance is the most natural human activity known to us, bringing with it many advantages – not the least being that it is the best and easiest way to meet, and make contact with, a member of the opposite sex. Among its many other benefits are that it:

* Is a wonderful, gentle but thorough way to exercise your body;
* Develops co-ordination of mind and muscle;
* Encourages good poise, regardless of age;
* Tones up the body and gives that "good-to-be-alive" feeling;
* Teaches the social graces;
* Helps to keep you youthful and up-to-date;
* Is one of the few hobbies that couples or friends can do together;
* Is a great social asset;
* Promotes confidence and self-assurance;
* Is probably the cheapest and most rewarding way to spend your leisure time;
* Can be started at five years of age and can still be enjoyed when you are 95!

A Brief History

Ballroom dancing, as we know it today, is made up of two distinct types of dances, namely "Modern" dances and "Latin" dances.

Modern dances were first on the scene, and owed much of their existence to a new sound that originated in America and was let loose on a startled world in the early years of the twentieth century. This new sound, of Afro-American origin, was called Ragtime.

The American dancing public reacted immediately to this exciting music by producing a variety of wild, strange dances with extraordinary names such as the Grizzly Bear, Turkey Trot, Bunny Hug, Shimmy, Black Bottom, and Charleston. The Charleston became for some time a dance craze, but these other dances soon dropped out of fashion.

Ragtime music, however, and the more sophisticated music styles that were to follow in the next few years, were to revolutionize completely the fundamental structure of social dancing throughout the world. Up to that time, French dancing masters taught dances based on the five foot positions used in classical ballet; Ragtime music heralded the start of "together" dancing based on a natural walking action.

The Modern Dances

During the period between 1920 and 1930, a group of British professionals developed four dances – English Waltz, Foxtrot, Quickstep, and Tango. These were suitable for the general public to dance in ballrooms to the popular music available at that time.

The English Waltz was so-named to distinguish it from The French (rotary) Waltz and the up-tempoed Viennese Waltz; instead of continuous turns, the British introduced diagonal patterns to construct their basic figures. The Foxtrot and The Quickstep were the offspring of a stage dance introduced by Harry Fox, an American. The modern Tango was based on an existing French version of the dance that was popular at the time. Along with The Viennese Waltz, a particular variation from Germany that was added later, these dances became collectively known as the Modern dances.

The Latin Dances

The first Afro-Cuban rhythm to become popular abroad was a Rumba. Cuban musicians, led by Don Azpiazu, introduced Rumba music to New York in 1929, and to Paris and London in 1930. Dancers on both sides of the Atlantic took a liking to this new dance, and within a few years The Square Rumba became the first Latin dance to be included in the West's social dance calendar. The basic figures used in this dance are in the form of a square – hence its name.

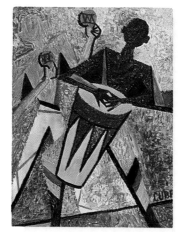

The arrival of The Rumba revived interest in other Latin dances, some of which had been introduced with little success years before, and by 1945 The Samba (from Brazil) and The Jive (from the US) became part of the social dance scene. The Paso Doble, based on a version of this dance from France, was also added to the Latin section in competitions, but it is not a favourite with social dancers.

In the late 1940s, three new Latin dance rhythms found their way from Cuba to the West; they were The Mambo, The Cha Cha Cha, and The Cuban Rumba.

The MAMBO was a fantastic success in the US during the early to mid-1950s, and it remains, to this day, what many Latin dancers call the national dance of the United States. Unfortunately, The MAMBO did not enjoy the same success in Europe – probably because good MAMBO music was not readily available. Consequently, The MAMBO still is not featured in international ballroom dance championships.

The CHA CHA CHA, however, was welcomed throughout the Western world and was, and still is, a great favourite with social dancers of all ages.

Pierre and Lavelle, two very well-known Latin dance teachers from London, were captivated by the simplicity of The CUBAN RUMBA (which, in later years, many said was a slow MAMBO). They saw it had great potential as a social dance and were convinced it would be far superior to The SQUARE RUMBA that was danced in the West at that time. But it took 14 years for The CUBAN RUMBA to replace the old SQUARE RUMBA.

Today, the ten ballroom dances that are the foundation of the social dance scene are the same ten standard dances used in international ballroom competitions and championships. They are The WALTZ, The QUICKSTEP, The FOXTROT, The TANGO, and The VIENNESE WALTZ in the Modern section and The RUMBA, The SAMBA, The CHA CHA CHA, The JIVE and The PASO DOBLE in the Latin section.

COMPETITION-STYLE DANCING

Of the millions of people throughout the world who regularly enjoy social dancing there are a number who are ultimately attracted to taking part in organized ballroom dance competitions.

Competition dancing is a form of ballroom dancing that has evolved from social dancing. It attracts people who love to dance and who have the urge to show their skill and talent in direct competition with other couples on the dance floor. Such people dance not only for their own satisfaction, but also to impress both the adjudicators who have been selected to decide who the best couples are and, of course, the audience. Competition dancing brings with it an element of show business and, consequently, additional factors to the quality of performance, musical interpretation, and characterization become important.

Many people are intrigued to know how judges of ballroom dance competitions decide which of the couples taking part should be awarded the winners' trophy. How do they make their choices? In fact, it is necessary for the judges of such events to have considerable knowledge and experience to make sound decisions.

The two most important facets of the dancers' performance that have to be assessed are quality and crowd appeal. Quality is expressed through the dancers' technique, musicality, and characterization; crowd appeal depends on the dancers' choreography, presentation, and personalities.

The standard of performance, therefore, is made up of many different elements taken together. Because individuals place a different value on each aspect, their assessments are subjective, so an uneven number of adjudicators is always used for major events. Additionally, a method of collating the judges' markings for each couple has been devised in which more weighting is given to the same and higher placings for each couple.

Because the two styles of ballroom dancing are so different, separate competitions are held for the Modern and Latin dances. The differences are particularly reflected by the costumes worn by the dancers during these competitions, and this is shown in the pages of THE BALLROOM DANCE PACK. Dresses worn for the Modern dances are long and flowing, to enhance the movements created during these dances. In contrast, the dresses worn for the Latin dances are designed to show the movements of the individual body parts used to interpret the various Latin rhythms.

Men wear formal full dress – white tie and tails – in the Modern section and soft, shirt-style tops, together with well-cut trousers, for the Latin section. Readers should refer to the section entitled WHAT SHALL I WEAR? at the back of the book for some pointers on proper dress for the dance floor.

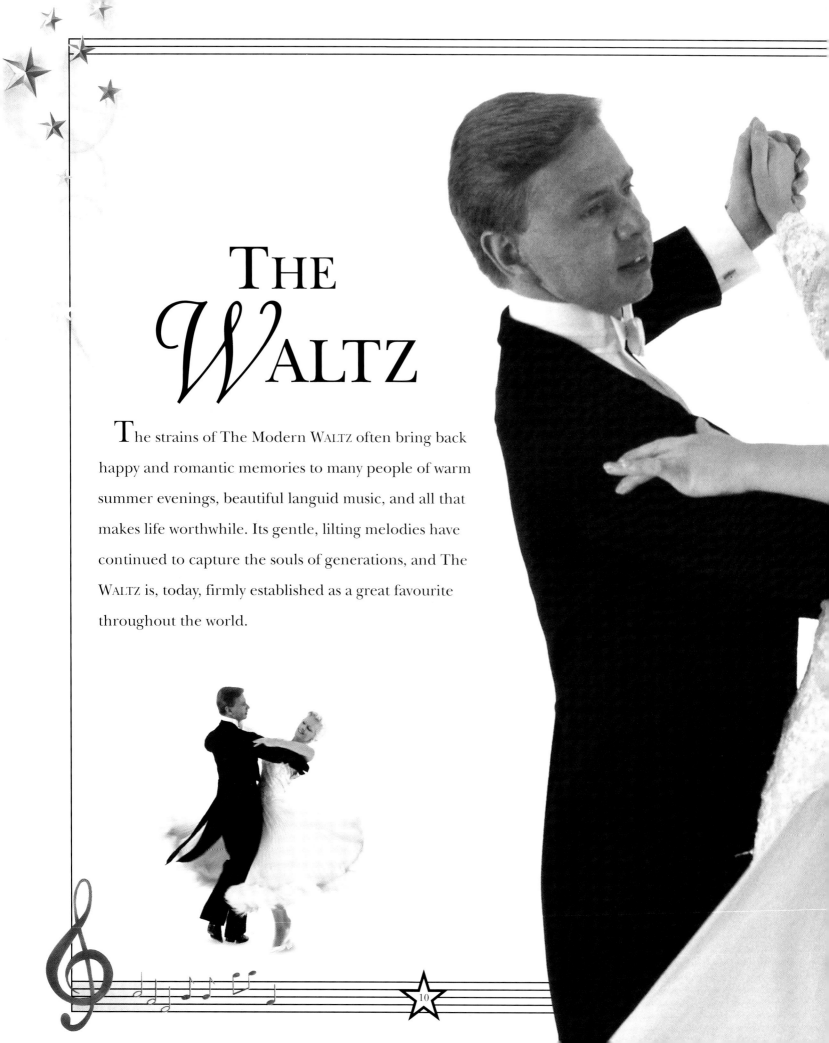

THE WALTZ

The strains of The Modern WALTZ often bring back happy and romantic memories to many people of warm summer evenings, beautiful languid music, and all that makes life worthwhile. Its gentle, lilting melodies have continued to capture the souls of generations, and The WALTZ is, today, firmly established as a great favourite throughout the world.

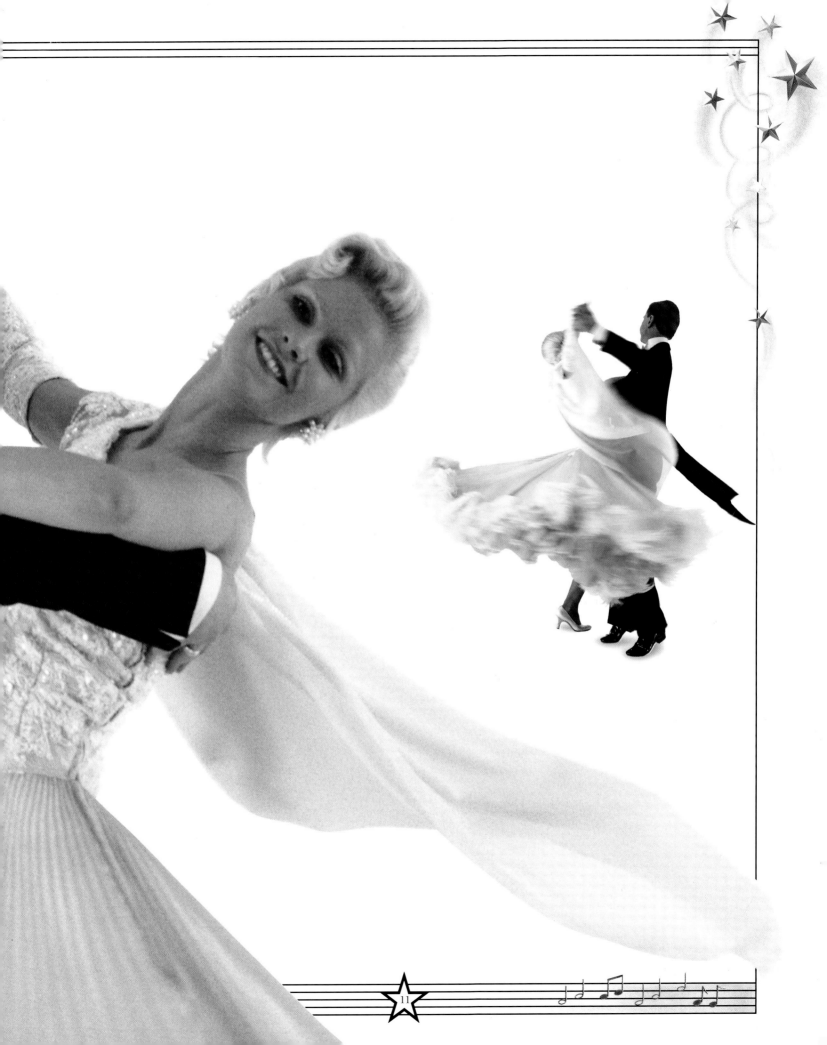

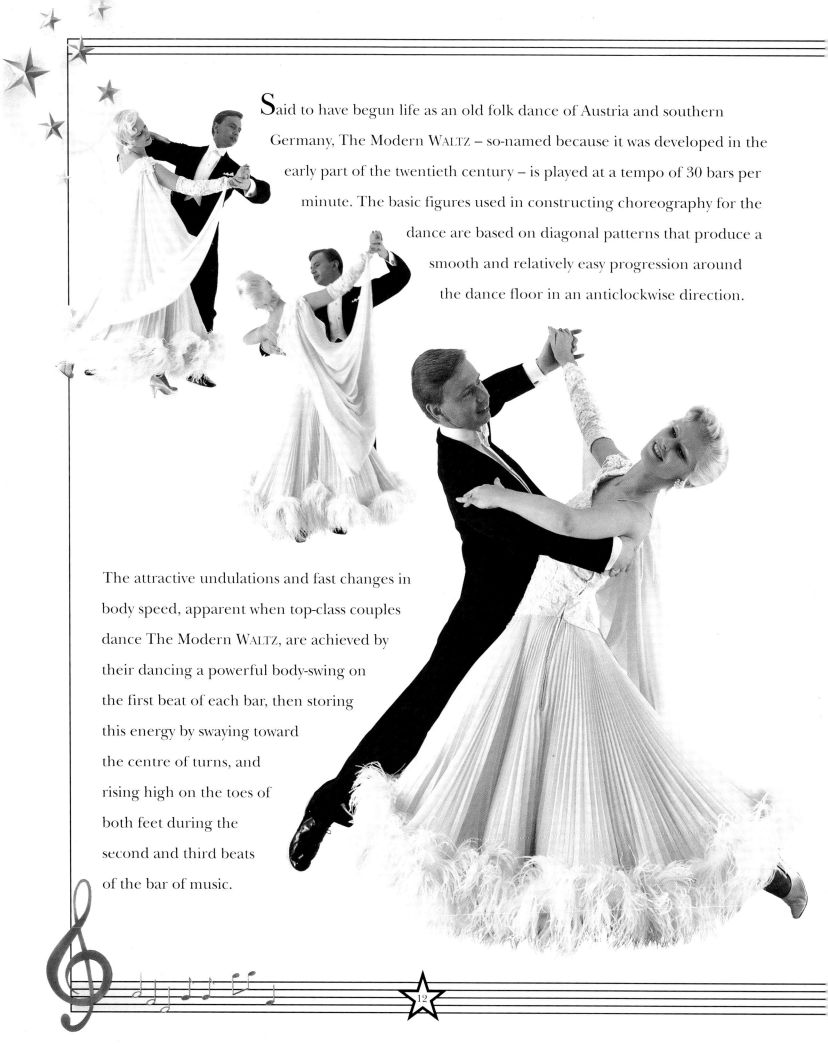

Said to have begun life as an old folk dance of Austria and southern Germany, The Modern WALTZ – so-named because it was developed in the early part of the twentieth century – is played at a tempo of 30 bars per minute. The basic figures used in constructing choreography for the dance are based on diagonal patterns that produce a smooth and relatively easy progression around the dance floor in an anticlockwise direction.

The attractive undulations and fast changes in body speed, apparent when top-class couples dance The Modern WALTZ, are achieved by their dancing a powerful body-swing on the first beat of each bar, then storing this energy by swaying toward the centre of turns, and rising high on the toes of both feet during the second and third beats of the bar of music.

A competition dancer requires a fit body and strong ankles to produce a good characterization of The Modern WALTZ in order to achieve considerable success in major international championships.

The Modern WALTZ is usually the first dance taught to beginners in dance schools. The simple construction of the basic figures, the regular, even changes of weight required throughout the dance, and the slow tempo – coupled with the easy-to-hear, repetitive, unsyncopated basic rhythm – are ideally suited to put beginners at ease and help them gain confidence.

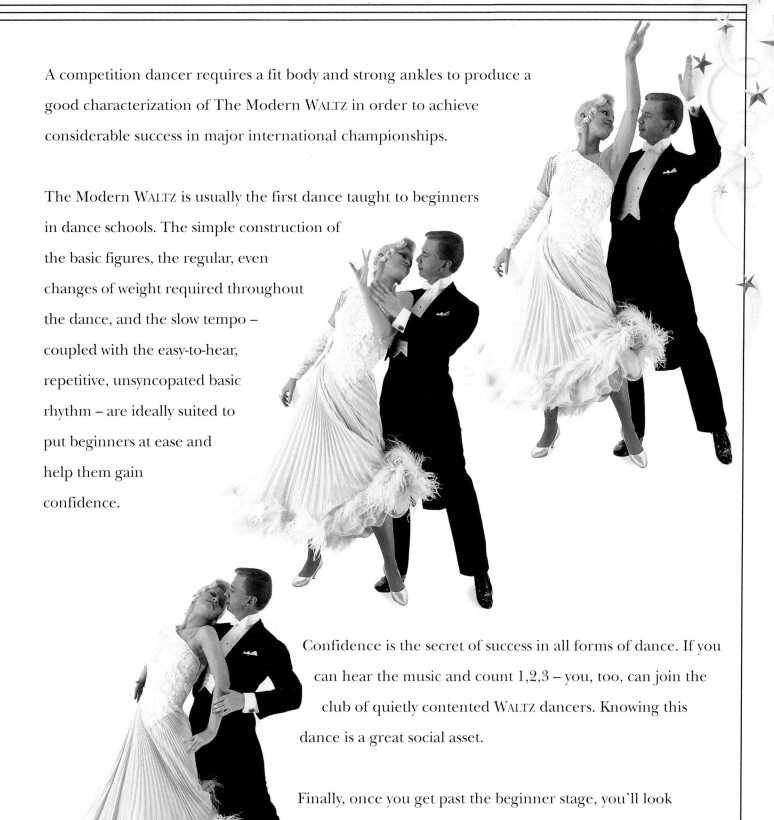

Confidence is the secret of success in all forms of dance. If you can hear the music and count 1,2,3 – you, too, can join the club of quietly contented WALTZ dancers. Knowing this dance is a great social asset.

Finally, once you get past the beginner stage, you'll look particularly good dancing The WALTZ if you and your partner are beautifully groomed and formally dressed.

MAN'S SOLO EXERCISE

Begin with feet together, weight on LF, facing in any direction, arms held slightly forward in a comfortable position. Take the first step on the first beat of any bar of music. Repeat the SOLO EXERCISE *ad lib.*

COUNT "THREE"

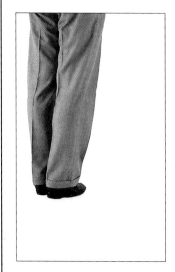

3 RF closed to LF

COUNT "TWO"

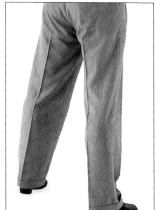

2 LF to side

COUNT "ONE"

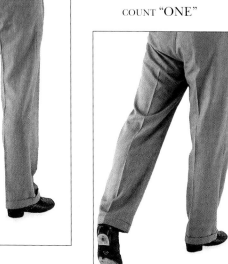

1 RF forward

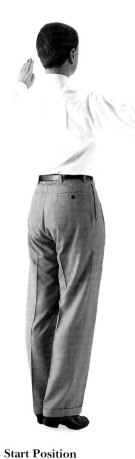

Start Position
M ~ Weight on LF, facing in any direction

COUNT "ONE"

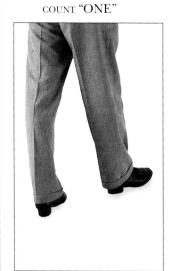

4 LF back

COUNT "TWO"

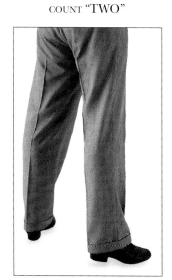

5 RF to side

COUNT "THREE"

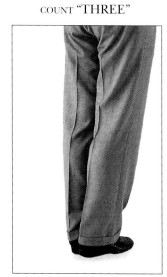

6 LF closed to RF

WOMAN'S SOLO EXERCISE

Begin with feet together, weight on RF, facing in any direction, arms held slightly forward in a comfortable position. Take the first step on the first beat of any bar of music. Repeat the SOLO EXERCISE *ad lib*.

COUNT "THREE"

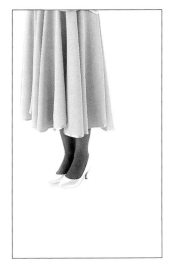

3 LF closed to RF

COUNT "TWO"

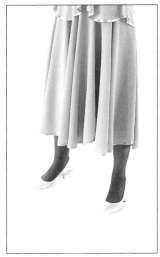

2 RF to side

COUNT "ONE"

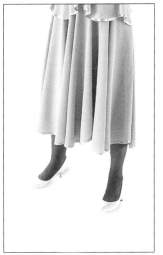

1 LF back

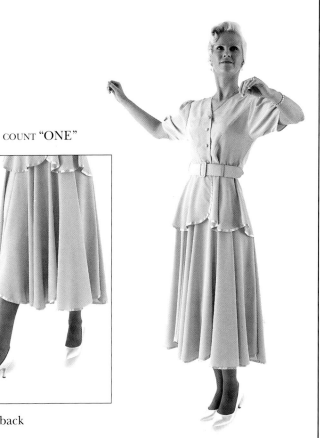

Start Position
W ~ Weight on RF, facing in any direction

COUNT "ONE"

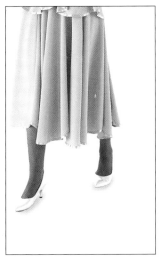

4 RF forward

COUNT "TWO"

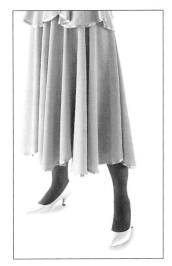

5 LF to side

COUNT "THREE"

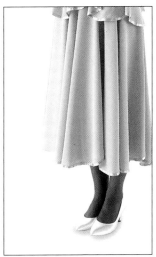

6 RF closed to LF

CLOSE HOLD

This is the normal stance for both fast and slow tempos. The arms can be held closer to the body if the dance floor is crowded.

MAN   **WOMAN**

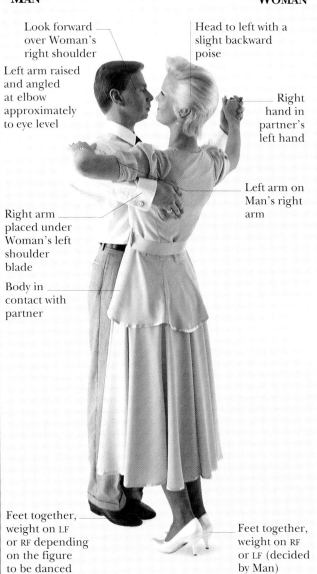

Look forward over Woman's right shoulder

Left arm raised and angled at elbow approximately to eye level

Right arm placed under Woman's left shoulder blade

Body in contact with partner

Feet together, weight on LF or RF depending on the figure to be danced

Head to left with a slight backward poise

Right hand in partner's left hand

Left arm on Man's right arm

Feet together, weight on RF or LF (decided by Man)

☆

DANCING THE WALTZ

This is one of the simplest dances to learn; you can Waltz just by repeating the 12 steps of THE QUARTER TURNS *ad lib*. If you slightly adjust the amount of turn as you approach each corner, you will progress in an anticlockwise direction around the dance floor.

THE QUARTER TURNS

COUNT "ONE"   COUNT "TWO"

Begin in CLOSE HOLD (see Box, left), weight on LF (Woman RF), facing diagonally to wall.

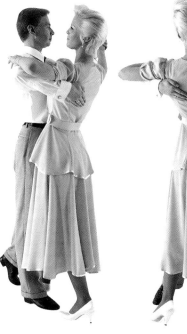

1 M ~ RF forward
W ~ LF back

2 M ~ LF to side
W ~ RF to side

COUNT "ONE"   COUNT "TWO"

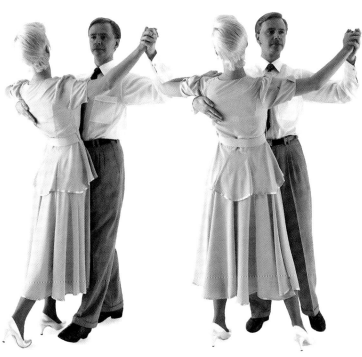

7 M ~ RF back
W ~ LF forward

8 M ~ LF to side
W ~ RF to side

COUNT "THREE"

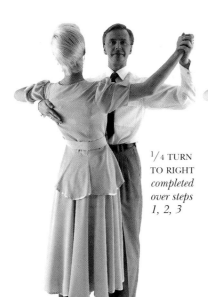

1/4 TURN TO RIGHT *completed over steps 1, 2, 3*

3 **M** ~ RF closed to LF
W ~ LF closed to RF

COUNT "ONE"

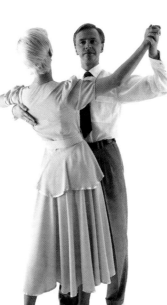

4 **M** ~ LF back
W ~ RF forward

COUNT "TWO"

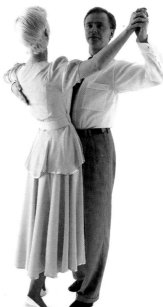

5 **M** ~ RF diagonally back
W ~ LF diagonally forward

COUNT "THREE"

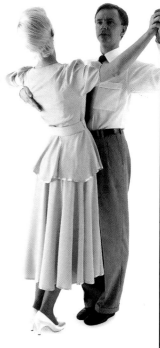

6 **M** ~ LF closed to RF
W ~ RF closed to LF

* Repeat *ad lib* or continue with THE NATURAL TURN

COUNT "THREE"

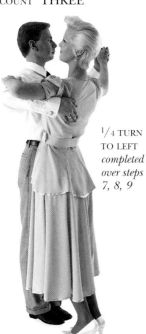

1/4 TURN TO LEFT *completed over steps 7, 8, 9*

9 **M** ~ RF closed to LF
W ~ LF closed to RF

COUNT "ONE"

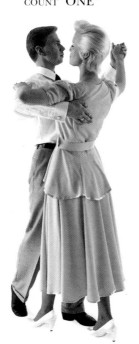

10 **M** ~ LF forward
W ~ RF back

COUNT "TWO"

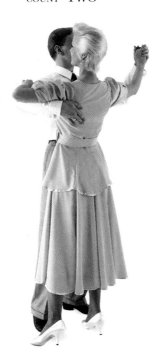

11 **M** ~ RF to side
W ~ LF to side

COUNT "THREE"

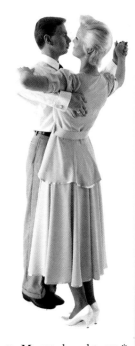

12 **M** ~ LF closed to RF *
W ~ RF closed to LF *

THE NATURAL TURN
Begin in CLOSE HOLD (see Box, p.16), weight on LF (Woman RF), facing diagonally to wall.

COUNT "ONE" COUNT "TWO" COUNT "THREE" COUNT "ONE" COUNT "TWO"

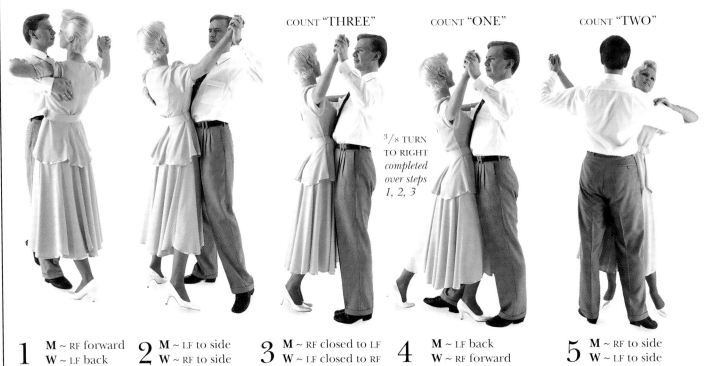

³/8 TURN TO RIGHT *completed over steps 1, 2, 3*

1 **M** ~ RF forward
W ~ LF back

2 **M** ~ LF to side
W ~ RF to side

3 **M** ~ RF closed to LF
W ~ LF closed to RF

4 **M** ~ LF back
W ~ RF forward

5 **M** ~ RF to side
W ~ LF to side

THE REVERSE TURN
Begin in CLOSE HOLD (see Box, p.16), weight on RF (Woman LF), facing diagonally to centre.

COUNT "ONE" COUNT "TWO" COUNT "THREE" COUNT "ONE" COUNT "TWO"

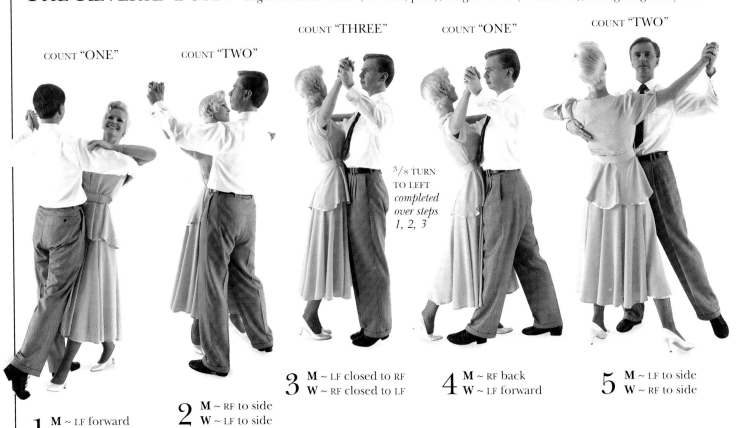

³/8 TURN TO LEFT *completed over steps 1, 2, 3*

1 **M** ~ LF forward
W ~ RF back

2 **M** ~ RF to side
W ~ LF to side

3 **M** ~ LF closed to RF
W ~ RF closed to LF

4 **M** ~ RF back
W ~ LF forward

5 **M** ~ LF to side
W ~ RF to side

THE FORWARD CHANGE (RLR)

Begin in CLOSE HOLD, weight on LF (Woman RF), facing diagonally to centre.

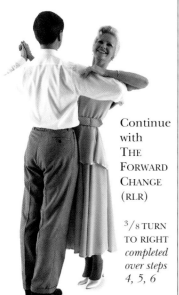

COUNT "THREE"

Continue
with
THE
FORWARD
CHANGE
(RLR)

3/8 TURN
TO RIGHT
*completed
over steps
4, 5, 6*

6 **M** ~ LF closed to RF
W ~ RF closed to LF

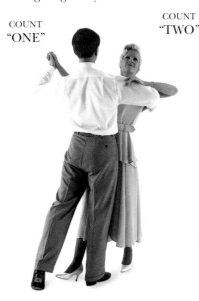

COUNT
"ONE"

COUNT
"TWO"

1 **M** ~ RF forward
W ~ LF back

2 **M** ~ LF to side
W ~ RF to side

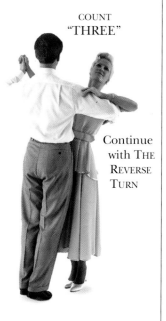

COUNT
"THREE"

Continue
with THE
REVERSE
TURN

3 **M** ~ RF closed to LF
W ~ LF closed to RF

THE FORWARD CHANGE (LRL)

Begin in CLOSE HOLD, weight on RF (Woman LF), facing diagonally to wall.

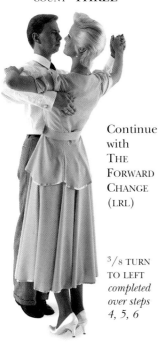

COUNT "THREE"

Continue
with
THE
FORWARD
CHANGE
(LRL)

3/8 TURN
TO LEFT
*completed
over steps
4, 5, 6*

6 **M** ~ RF closed to LF
W ~ LF closed to RF

COUNT "ONE"

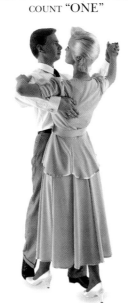

COUNT "TWO"

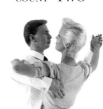
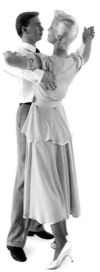

1 **M** ~ LF forward
W ~ RF back

2 **M** ~ RF to side
W ~ LF to side

COUNT "THREE"

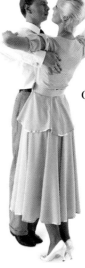

Continue
with
1) THE
NATURAL
TURN
or
2) THE
QUARTER
TURNS

3 **M** ~ LF closed to RF
W ~ RF closed to LF

The QUICKSTEP

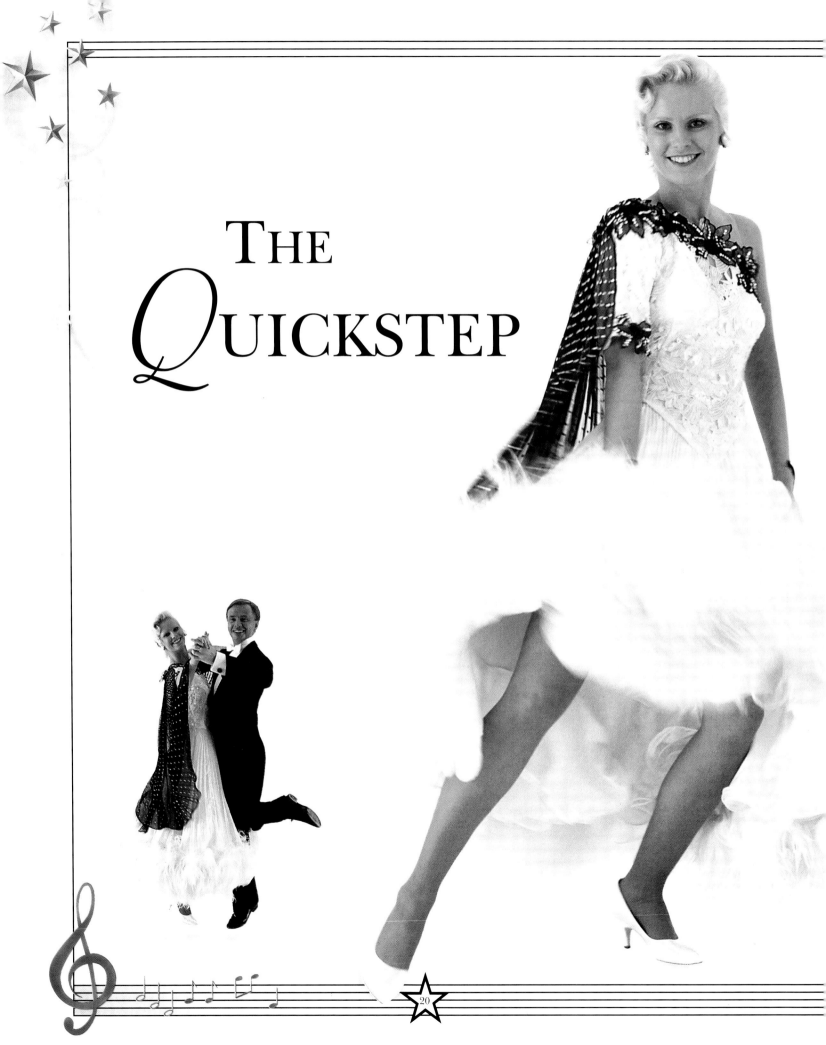

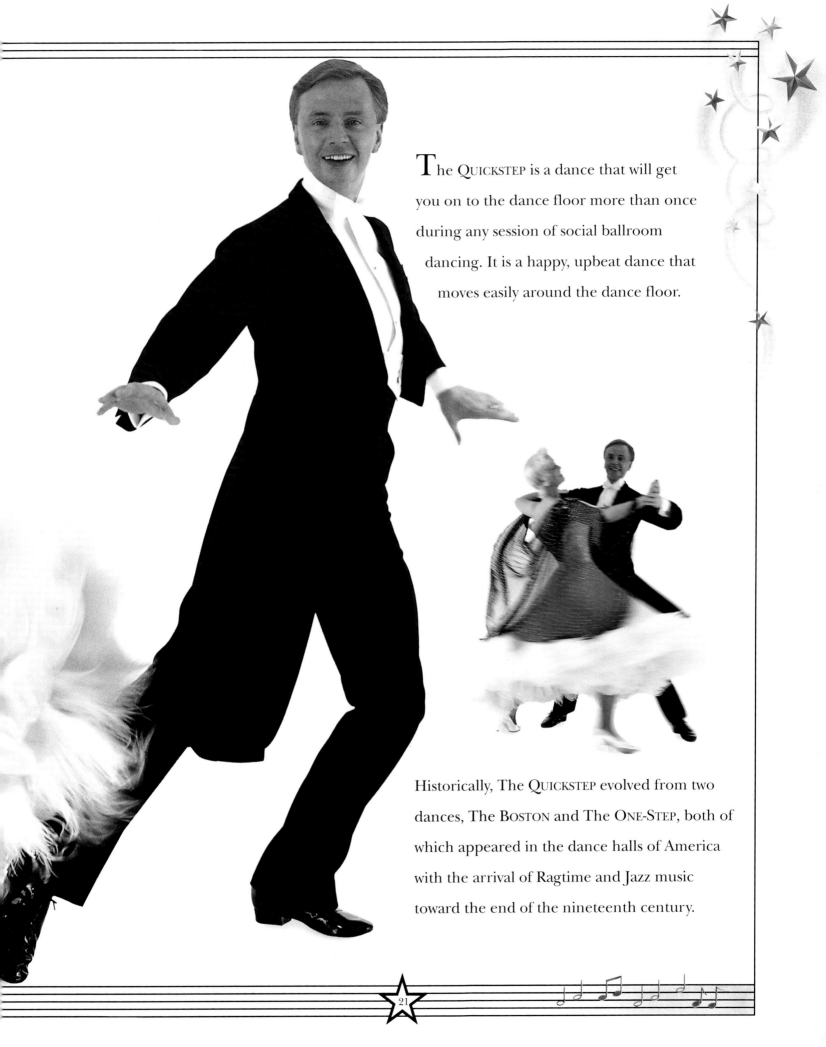

The QUICKSTEP is a dance that will get you on to the dance floor more than once during any session of social ballroom dancing. It is a happy, upbeat dance that moves easily around the dance floor.

Historically, The QUICKSTEP evolved from two dances, The BOSTON and The ONE-STEP, both of which appeared in the dance halls of America with the arrival of Ragtime and Jazz music toward the end of the nineteenth century.

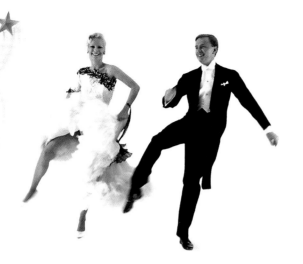 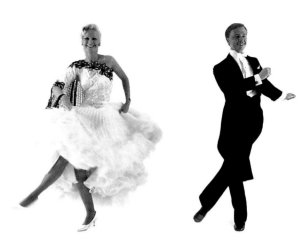

This exciting new music had a profound effect on social dancing styles. Dancers turned their backs on dances based on the five foot positions of classical ballet, during which everyone danced the same sequence, and turned to those that used normal walking steps.

The BOSTON and The ONE-STEP were the first two dances based on a forward step (or number of steps), using a heel lead followed by two or more, forward steps on the balls of the feet. (Later, these steps were sometimes replaced by crossing one foot behind the other [Lock Steps]). These two dances were followed in the 1920s by The QUICKSTEP, which was one of the standard ballroom dances developed to interpret the more sophisticated, up-tempo music.

Bright music, tricky steps, a light and happy mood – that's The QUICKSTEP. It is a moving dance based on Walks and Chassés that fit easily to the four-in-the-bar music. Like The WALTZ, diagonal patterns are used for its basic figures. The standardized tempo is 50 bars per minute.

Because the tempo of the music is relatively fast, thinking time is at a premium; be sure that you are familiar with

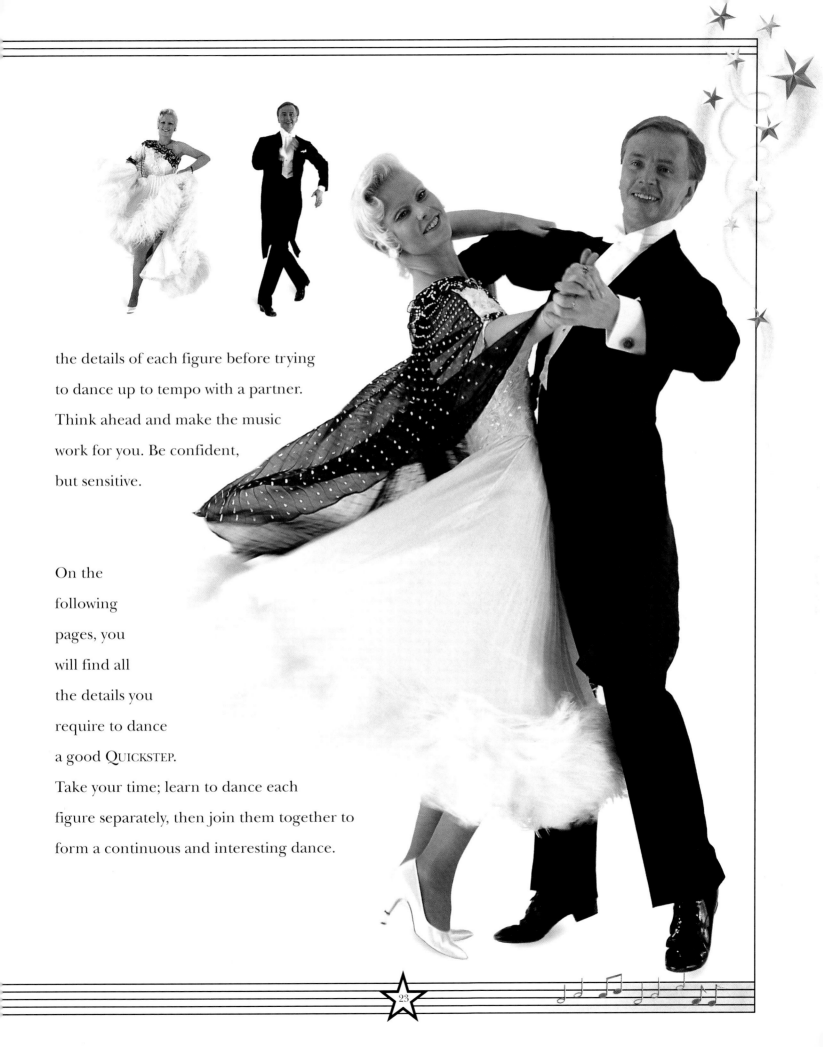

the details of each figure before trying

to dance up to tempo with a partner.

Think ahead and make the music

work for you. Be confident,

but sensitive.

On the

following

pages, you

will find all

the details you

require to dance

a good QUICKSTEP.

Take your time; learn to dance each

figure separately, then join them together to

form a continuous and interesting dance.

SOLO EXERCISE

The object of this exercise is to help you master the weight changes and timing required when dancing chassés – a movement used in many QUICKSTEP figures.

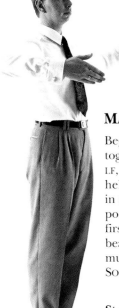

MAN

Begin with feet together, weight on LF, facing wall, arms held slightly forward in a comfortable position. Take the first step on the first beat of any bar of music. Repeat the SOLO EXERCISE *ad lib*.

Start Position
Weight on LF, facing wall

COUNT "SLOW"

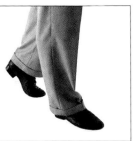

1 RF forward

COUNT "QUICK"

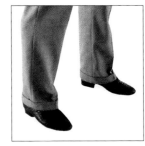

2 LF to side

COUNT "SLOW"

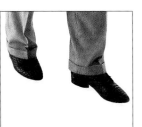

5 RF back

COUNT "QUICK"

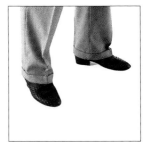

6 LF to side

WOMAN

Begin with feet together, weight on RF, backing wall, arms held slightly forward in a comfortable position. Take the first step on the first beat of any bar of music. Repeat the SOLO EXERCISE *ad lib*.

Start Position
Weight on RF, backing wall

COUNT "SLOW"

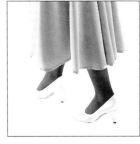

1 LF back

COUNT "QUICK"

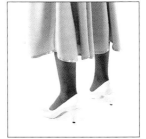

2 RF to side

COUNT "SLOW"

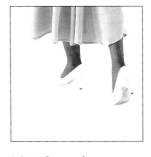

5 LF forward

COUNT "QUICK"

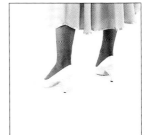

6 RF to side

COUNT "QUICK"   COUNT "SLOW"

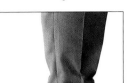 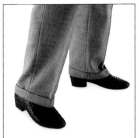

3 RF closed to LF   **4** LF to side

COUNT "QUICK"   COUNT "SLOW"

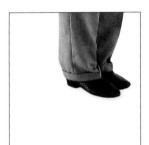

7 RF closed to LF   **8** LF to side

COUNT "QUICK"   COUNT "SLOW"

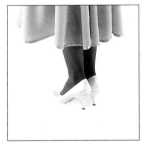 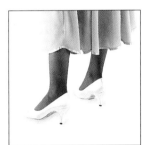

3 LF closed to RF   **4** RF to side

COUNT "QUICK"   COUNT "SLOW"

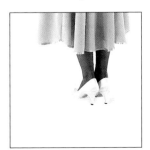 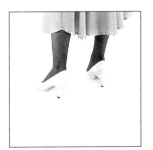

7 LF closed to RF   **8** RF to side

CLOSE HOLD

This is the start position for most of The QUICKSTEP figures shown on the following pages. It is exactly the same hold as for The WALTZ.

MAN   **WOMAN**

Look forward over the Woman's right shoulder

Head to left with a slight backward poise

Left arm raised and angled at elbow approximately to eye level

Right hand in partner's left hand

Right arm placed under Woman's left shoulder blade

Left arm on Man's right arm

Body in contact with partner

Feet together, weight on LF or RF, depending on the figure to be danced

Feet together, weight on RF or LF (decided by Man)

THE QUARTER TURNS

Begin in CLOSE HOLD (see Box, p.25) weight on LF (Woman RF), facing diagonally to wall.

COUNT "SLOW"   COUNT "QUICK"   COUNT "QUICK"   COUNT "SLOW"

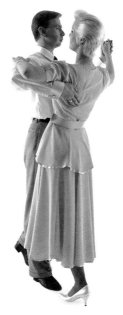 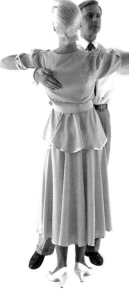 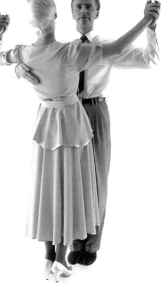 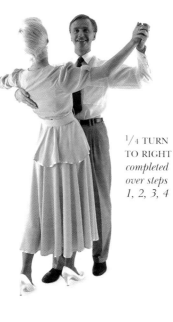

¼ TURN TO RIGHT completed over steps 1, 2, 3, 4

1   **M** ~ RF forward
W ~ LF back

2   **M** ~ LF to side
W ~ RF to side

3   **M** ~ RF closed to LF
W ~ LF closed to RF

4   **M** ~ LF to side and slightly back
W ~ RF diagonally forward

THE PROMENADE CHASSÉ

Begin in CLOSE HOLD, weight on LF (Woman RF), backing diagonally to centre having danced steps 1 to 4 of THE QUARTER TURNS.

COUNT "SLOW"   COUNT "QUICK"   COUNT "QUICK"   COUNT "SLOW"

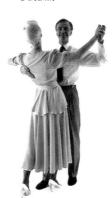 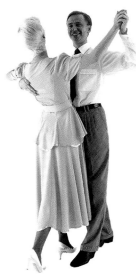 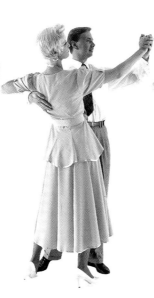 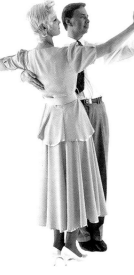 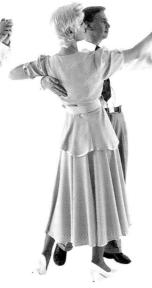

Start Position
Weight on LF (Woman RF), backing diagonally to centre

1   **M** ~ RF back
W ~ LF forward

2   **M** ~ LF to side in PP
W ~ RF to side in PP

3   **M** ~ RF closed to LF
W ~ LF closed to RF

4   **M** ~ LF to side in PP
W ~ RF to side in PP

COUNT "SLOW"   COUNT "QUICK"   COUNT "QUICK"   COUNT "SLOW"

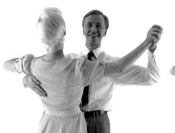
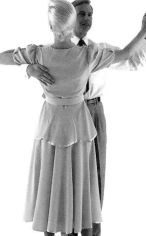
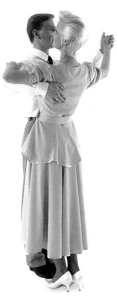
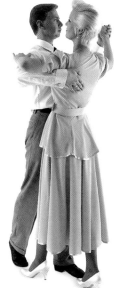

Repeat *ad lib,*
or continue
with steps
1 to 4 of THE
QUARTER TURNS,
followed by
THE PROMENADE
CHASSÉ

¹/₄ TURN
TO LEFT
*completed
over steps
5, 6, 7, 8*

5 **M** ~ RF back
W ~ LF forward

6 **M** ~ LF to side
(small step)
W ~ RF to side

7 **M** ~ RF closed to LF
W ~ LF closed to RF

8 **M** ~ LF forward
W ~ RF back

COUNT "SLOW"   COUNT "QUICK"   COUNT "QUICK"   COUNT "SLOW"

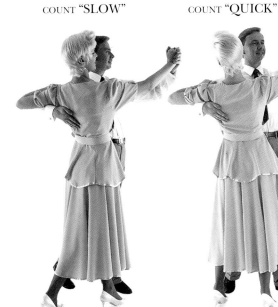
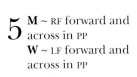
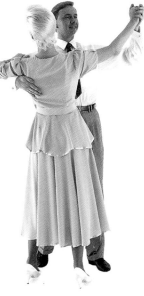
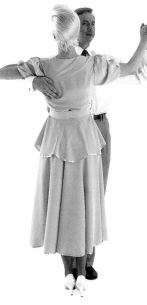
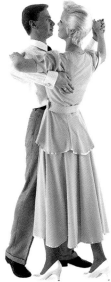

Continue with
1) THE QUARTER
TURNS, begun
RF forward
outside Woman,
or
2) THE LOCK STEP

5 **M** ~ RF forward and
across in PP
W ~ LF forward and
across in PP

6 **M** ~ LF to side
W ~ RF to side,
turning to left

7 **M** ~ RF closed to LF
W ~ LF closed to RF,
turning to face Man

8 **M** ~ LF to side and slightly
forward, preparing to step
outside Woman
W ~ RF to side and slightly
back

THE LOCK STEP

Begin in CLOSE HOLD, weight on LF (Woman RF), preparing to step outside partner having danced THE PROMENADE CHASSÉ.

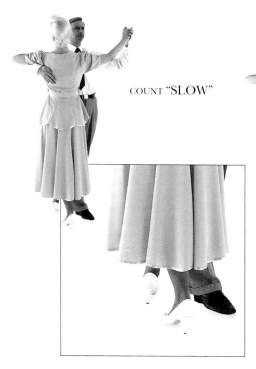

COUNT "SLOW"

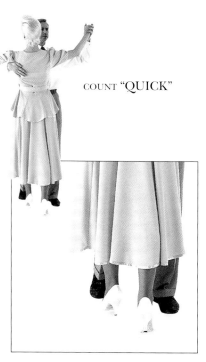

COUNT "QUICK"

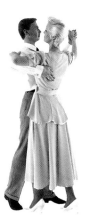

Start Position
Weight on LF (Woman RF), preparing to step outside partner

1 **M** ~ RF forward outside Woman
W ~ LF back, Man outside

2 **M** ~ LF forward (left shoulder leading *)
W ~ RF back (right shoulder leading *)

THE NATURAL PIVOT TURN

Begin in CLOSE HOLD (see Box, p.25), weight on LF (Woman RF), facing diagonally to wall near a corner.

COUNT "SLOW"

COUNT "QUICK"

COUNT "QUICK"

Dance this figure to turn a corner of the dance floor. After step 4, you will be facing diagonally to the wall of the new LOD with the RF held forward without weight (Woman LF held back without weight).

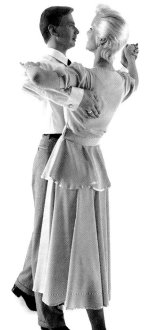

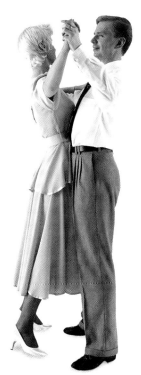

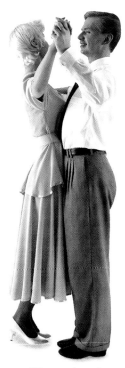

1 **M** ~ RF forward
W ~ LF back

2 **M** ~ LF to side
W ~ RF to side

3 **M** ~ RF closed to LF
W ~ LF closed to RF

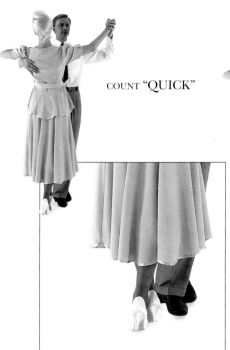

COUNT "QUICK"

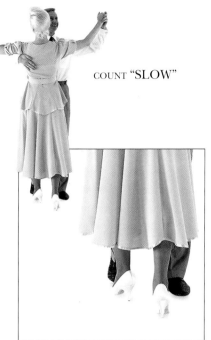

COUNT "SLOW"

* LEFT SHOULDER LEADING
In this figure the Man must step forward outside his partner without losing body contact. To facilitate this movement, he turns his body slightly to the right. The Woman will follow by turning her body slightly to the right. Steps forward outside the partner can then be made without loss of body contact – hence the dance term "left shoulder leading".

Continue with
1) THE QUARTER TURNS
or, at a corner,
2) THE NATURAL PIVOT TURN, both begun RF forward outside the Woman on her right side

3 **M** ~ RF crossed behind LF
W ~ LF crossed in front of RF

4 **M** ~ LF forward and slightly to side, preparing to step outside Woman
W ~ RF back and slightly to side

COUNT "SLOW"

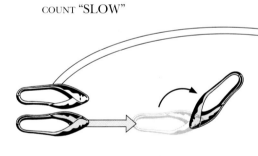

LF without weight

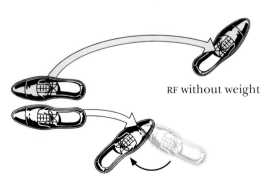

RF without weight

** HOW TO DANCE THE PIVOT
M ~ LF back, then turn $^3/_8$ to RIGHT, on ball of LF, retaining RF forward in front of body without weight
W ~ RF forward, then turn $^3/_8$ to RIGHT on ball of RF, retaining LF back and slightly to side without weight

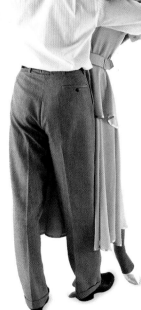

Continue with
1) THE QUARTER TURNS or
2) any QUICKSTEP figures that begin with RF (Woman LF), from facing diagonally to wall of new LOD.

4 **M** ~ LF back, then pivot **
W ~ RF forward, then pivot **

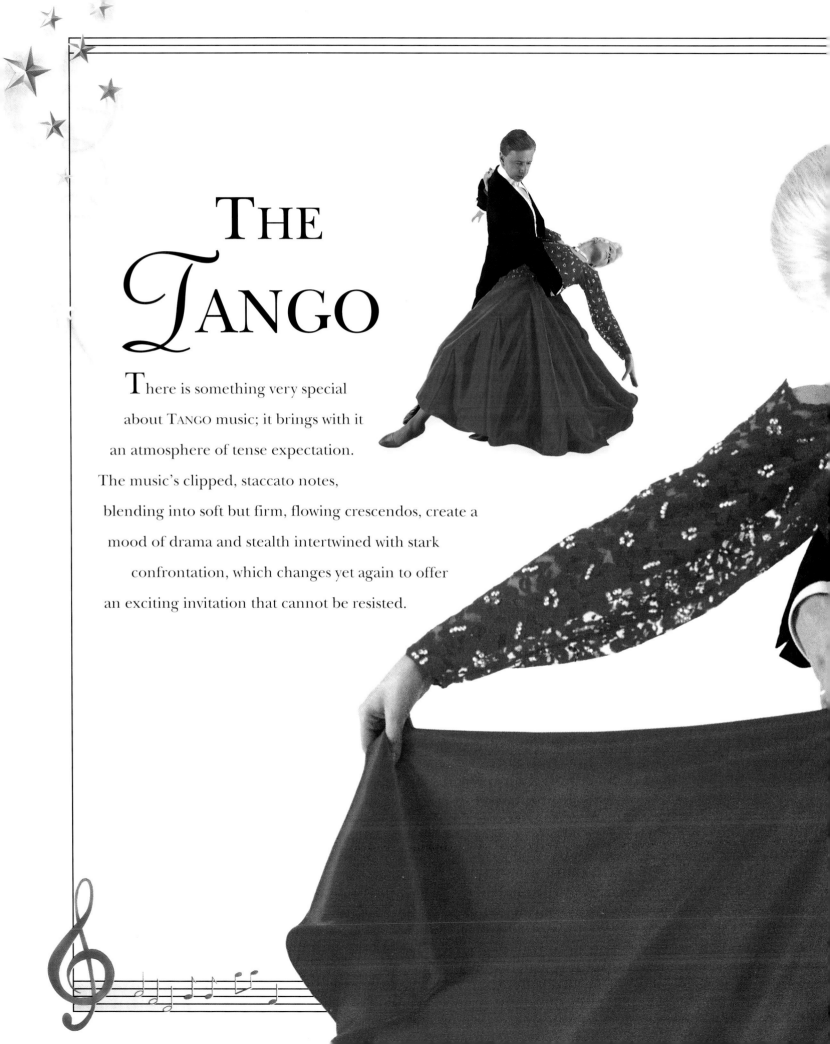

THE TANGO

There is something very special
about TANGO music; it brings with it
an atmosphere of tense expectation.
The music's clipped, staccato notes,
blending into soft but firm, flowing crescendos, create a
mood of drama and stealth intertwined with stark
confrontation, which changes yet again to offer
an exciting invitation that cannot be resisted.

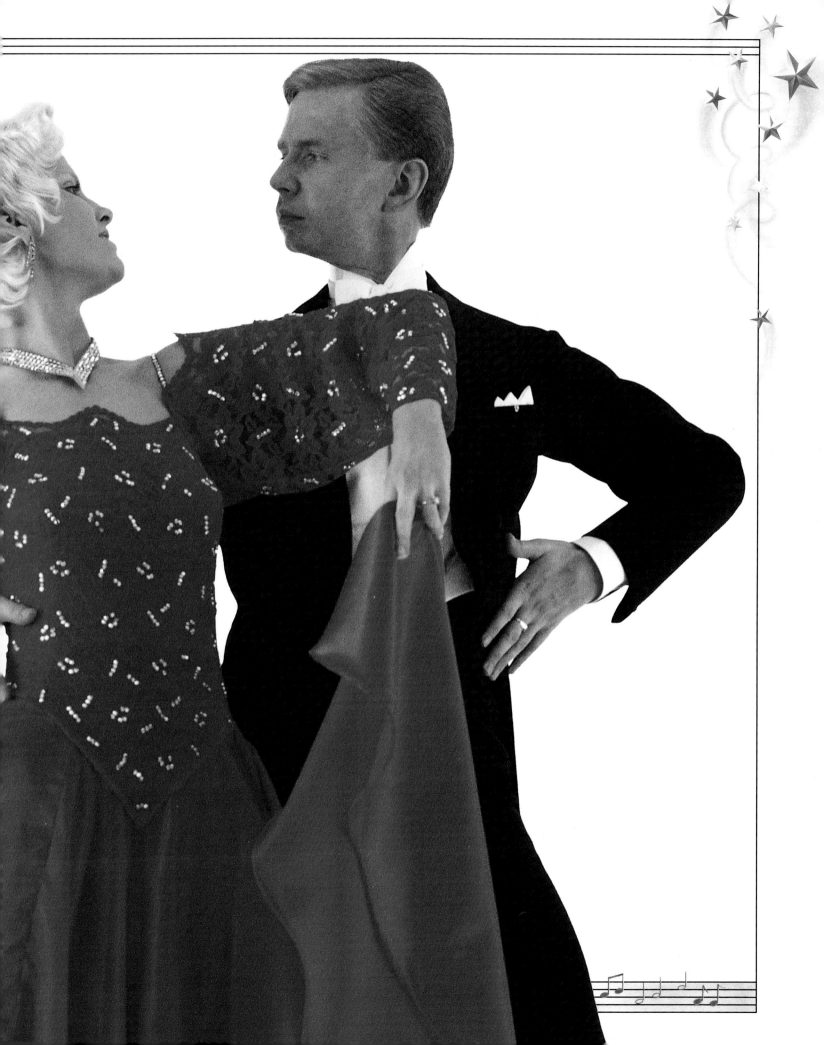

The dance, handed down by generations of TANGO dancers, originated in the slums and backstreets of Argentina and for over 100 years was considered too immodest for the dance halls. Cleaned up, it became fashionable in Europe in the early 1900s. Surprisingly, it is not a difficult dance to learn; the basic figures are easy to master. The secret of capturing the drama of The TANGO, however, lies in taking up the correct posture and hold, and achieving the elusive cat-like movement used during each Walk.

It is important to pay strict attention to the relative positions of your bodies when taking up The TANGO's Close Hold position. Dancers should note carefully the man's right shoulder lead, and that each time his feet are closed, the ball of his right foot is brought to the instep of his left foot (*vice versa* for the woman [see Box, p.35]).

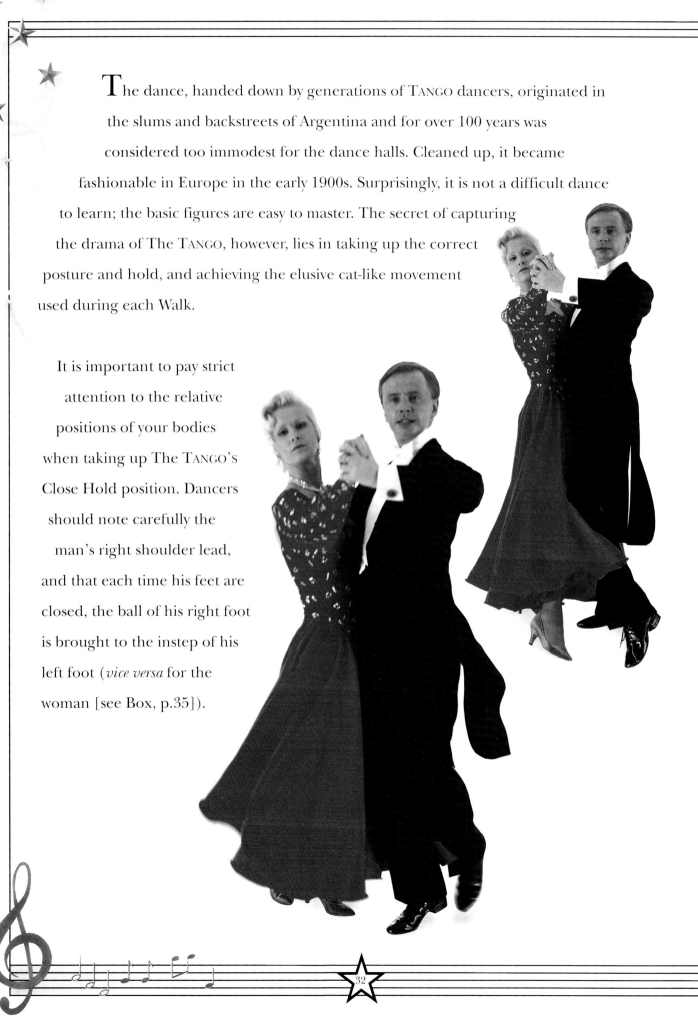

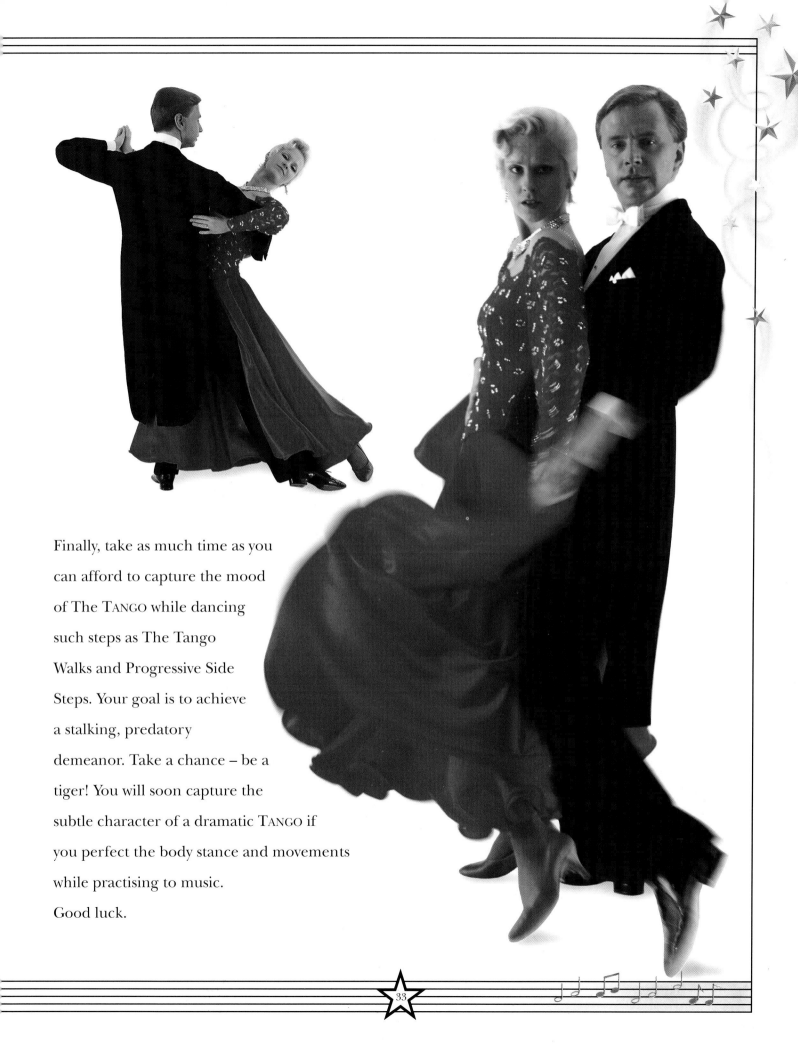

Finally, take as much time as you can afford to capture the mood of The TANGO while dancing such steps as The Tango Walks and Progressive Side Steps. Your goal is to achieve a stalking, predatory demeanor. Take a chance – be a tiger! You will soon capture the subtle character of a dramatic TANGO if you perfect the body stance and movements while practising to music. Good luck.

SOLO EXERCISE

Correctly danced TANGO WALKS will help to
achieve the character and mood of the
dance. Body positions resulting from the
CLOSE HOLD used for The TANGO produce
WALKS with unusual foot positions. These
require practise, hence this SOLO EXERCISE.
When TANGO WALKS are repeated *ad lib* they
trace out a circle approximately 3 meters
(10 feet) in diameter – see diagram.

To start the SOLO EXERCISE begin with the
feet together, weight on RF (Woman LF); see
CLOSE HOLD on opposite page for the
correct position for the feet, knees, and
body. Take the first step on the first beat of
any bar of music. Repeat SOLO EXERCISE
ad lib.

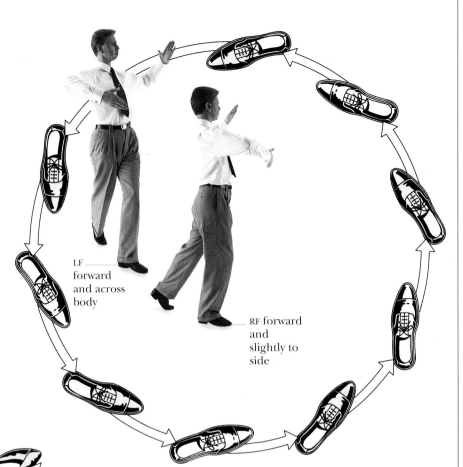

LF forward and across body

RF forward and slightly to side

MAN

Step forward with LF to finish forward and across
body, for the count of "SLOW"; when the LF is in
position, allow the right knee and ankle to flex,
retaining both feet in position. It is helpful to use
a count of "and" for this knee-and-ankle action.
The complete WALK will take the time of one
count of "SLOW".

To continue, step forward with RF to finish
forward and slightly to side for the count of
"SLOW", then repeat the same knee-and-
ankle flexing action described above. This
second completed WALK will take the time
of one count of "SLOW". Repeat these two
steps *ad lib*.

RF back under body

LF back and slightly to side

WOMAN

Step back with RF to finish back under body,
without lowering right heel, for the count of
"SLOW". Lower heel of RF. It is helpful to use a
count of "and" for this lowering action. The
completed WALK will take the time of one count
of "SLOW".

To continue, step back with LF to finish back and
slightly to side, without lowering left heel, for the
count of "SLOW"; then lower left heel as described
above. This second complete WALK will take the time
of one count of "SLOW". Repeat these two steps
ad lib.

CLOSE HOLD

To capture the magic of The TANGO, it is necessary to spend time learning to look right – even before you start to move. Study the photographs below. Note that the right shoulder should lead; this is achieved by angling the whole body over the feet so that when the feet are closed, the ball of the RF is closed to the instep of the LF with both knees slightly compressed. (The Woman closes instep of LF to ball of RF.) Note also the more compact hold; the Man's right arm moves further across the Woman's back and the Woman's left arm and hand touch her partner's body just under his right arm.

WOMAN

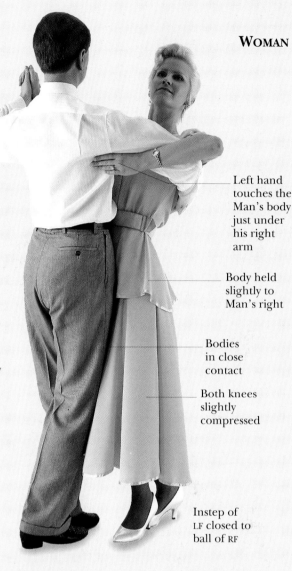

Left hand touches the Man's body just under his right arm

Body held slightly to Man's right

Bodies in close contact

Both knees slightly compressed

Instep of LF closed to ball of RF

MAN

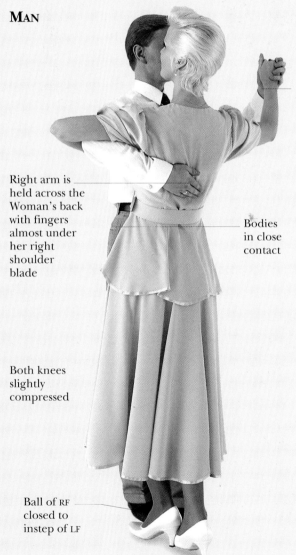

Left hand holds the Woman's right hand a little closer to the body and lower than in The WALTZ and The QUICKSTEP

Right arm is held across the Woman's back with fingers almost under her right shoulder blade

Bodies in close contact

Both knees slightly compressed

Ball of RF closed to instep of LF

TO ACHIEVE CLOSE HOLD

Stand directly in front of your partner, so that your bodies touch at hip level, with your feet together and parallel. The majority of weight is felt toward the front of each foot. Turn the whole body, in one piece, almost $1/8$ to LEFT by swivelling on both feet. After this turn the feet will still be parallel, but the ball of the RF will be level with the instep of the LF. (The Woman's left instep will be closed to the ball of her RF and she will have moved slightly to the Man's right.)

THE WALKS AND PROGRESSIVE SIDE STEP

Begin in CLOSE HOLD
(see Box, p.35), weight
on RF (Woman LF), facing
diagonally to wall.

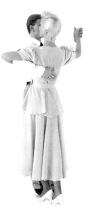

Start Position
Weight on RF (Woman
LF), facing diagonally
to wall

COUNT "SLOW"

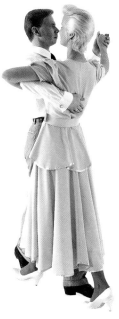

1 **M** ~ LF forward
W ~ RF back

COUNT "SLOW"

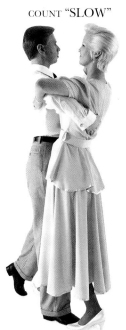

2 **M** ~ RF forward
W ~ LF back

COUNT "QUICK"

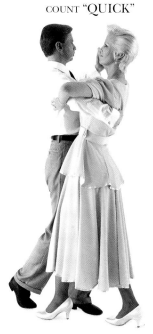

3 **M** ~ LF forward (short step)
W ~ RF back (short step)

THE REVERSE TURN

Begin in CLOSE HOLD,
weight on RF (Woman LF),
facing diagonally
to centre.

COUNT "QUICK"

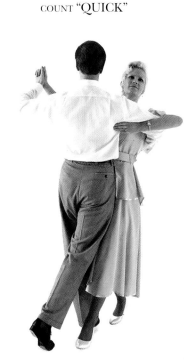

1 **M** ~ LF forward
W ~ RF back

COUNT "QUICK"

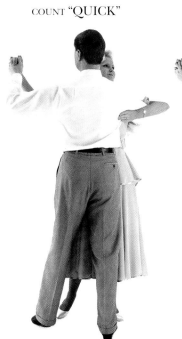

2 **M** ~ RF to side and slightly
back
W ~ LF to side and slightly
forward

COUNT "SLOW"

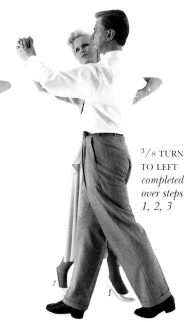

³/₈ TURN
TO LEFT
*completed
over steps
1, 2, 3*

3 **M** ~ LF back, Woman outside
W ~ RF forward, outside Man

COUNT "QUICK"

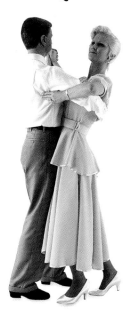

If you continue to dance this figure *ad lib* repeating from step 1, you will progress anticlockwise in a circle approximately 3-3¹/₂ meters (10-12 feet) in diameter.

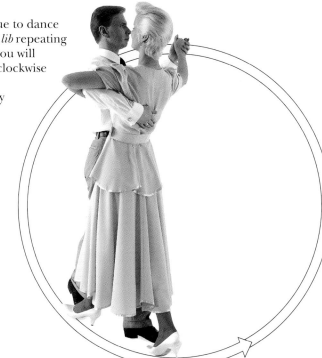

Continue with two WALKS – LF, RF (Woman RF, LF), finished facing diagonally to centre, then THE REVERSE TURN

4 **M** ~ RF to side and slightly back (short step)
W ~ LF to side and slightly forward (short step)

COUNT "QUICK"

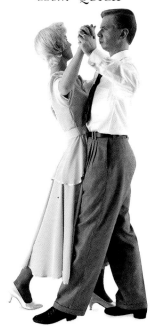

COUNT "QUICK"

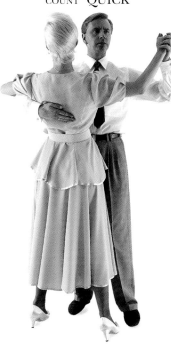

COUNT "SLOW"

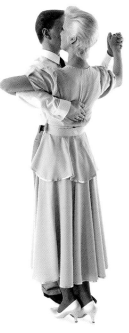

Continue with two WALKS – LF, RF (Woman RF, LF), then PROGRESSIVE LINK AND CLOSED PROMENADE

³/₈ TURN TO LEFT *completed over steps 4, 5, 6*

4 **M** ~ RF back
W ~ LF forward

5 **M** ~ LF to side and slightly forward
W ~ RF to side and slightly back

6 **M** ~ Ball of RF closed to instep of LF
W ~ Instep of LF closed to ball of RF

PROGRESSIVE LINK AND CLOSED PROMENADE

Begin in CLOSE HOLD, weight on RF (Woman LF), after two WALKS – LF, RF (Woman RF, LF), finished facing diagonally to wall.

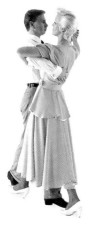

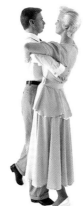

Dance two WALKS
Man ~ LF, RF
(Woman ~ RF, LF)

COUNT "QUICK"

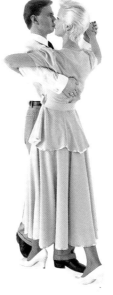

1 **M** ~ LF forward
W ~ RF back

COUNT "QUICK"

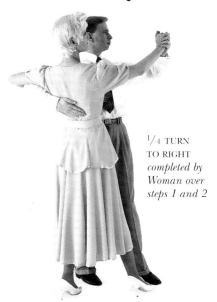

¹/₄ TURN TO RIGHT *completed by Woman over steps 1 and 2*

2 **M** ~ Turning body to RIGHT, RF to side and slightly back (short step). Release LEFT heel, moving LEFT knee toward RIGHT knee. You are now in PP.
W ~ Turning body to RIGHT, LF to side (short step). Release RIGHT heel, moving RIGHT knee toward LEFT knee. You are now in PP.

NATURAL ROCK TURN

Begin in CLOSE HOLD, weight on LF (Woman RF), having danced one WALK – LF (Woman RF), finished facing diagonally to wall.

COUNT "SLOW"

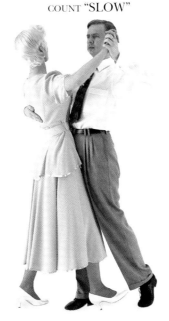

1 **M** ~ RF forward, turning to RIGHT
W ~ LF back, turning to RIGHT

COUNT "QUICK"

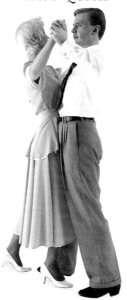

2 **M** ~ LF diagonally back
W ~ RF forward and slightly to side

COUNT "QUICK"

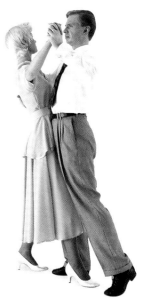

3 **M** ~ Transfer weight forward to RF
W ~ Moving LF slightly to LEFT, transfer weight back to LF

* Continue with one WALK – LF, then NATURAL ROCK TURN

COUNT "SLOW"   COUNT "QUICK"   COUNT "QUICK"   COUNT "SLOW"

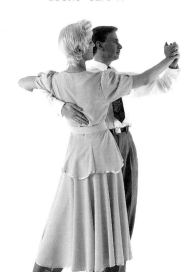 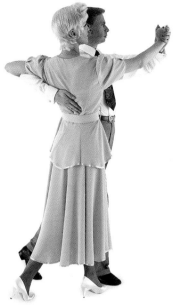 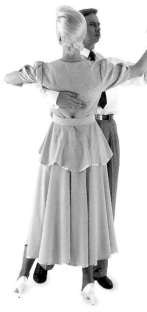 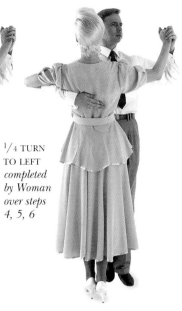

$\frac{1}{4}$ TURN
TO LEFT
*completed
by Woman
over steps
4, 5, 6*

3 M ~ LF to side in PP
W ~ RF to side in PP

4 M ~ RF forward and across in PP
W ~ LF forward and across in PP

5 M ~ LF to side and slightly forward
W ~ RF to side and slightly back

6 M ~ Ball of RF closed to instep of LF *
W ~ Instep of LF closed to ball of RF *

** Continue with THE WALKS AND PROGRESSIVE SIDE STEP

COUNT "SLOW"   COUNT "QUICK"   COUNT "QUICK"   COUNT "SLOW"

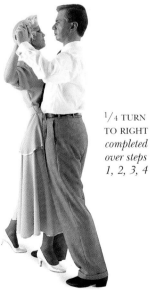 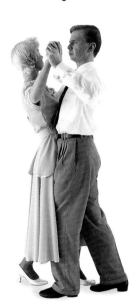 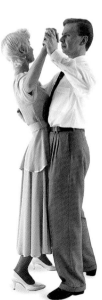 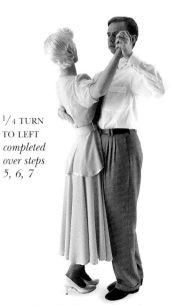

$\frac{1}{4}$ TURN
TO RIGHT
*completed
over steps
1, 2, 3, 4*

$\frac{1}{4}$ TURN
TO LEFT
*completed
over steps
5, 6, 7*

4 M ~ LF back (small step)
W ~ RF forward (small step)

5 M ~ RF back
W ~ LF forward

6 M ~ LF to side and slightly forward
W ~ RF to side and slightly back

7 M ~ Ball of RF closed to instep of LF **
W ~ Instep of LF closed to ball of RF **

THE CHA CHA CHA

Cheeky, gay, and carefree, The CHA CHA CHA is a together dance – one to do with your mother or sister as well as with your lover. Not so intimate as The TANGO or The RUMBA, it also is one of the easiest dances to learn. Beginners, both men and women, find its Latin rhythm easy to follow because the clearly marked beats can be counted out in time with the music. With social dancers throughout the world, it is a perennial favourite.

The dance is based on a Chassé movement (three linked steps), which is danced to coincide with the accented beats in each bar of the music. The name CHA CHA CHA is said to represent the sound made by the feet of the dancers on the floor when they dance this chassé.

When I was defending my World Championship titles – now more years ago than I care to recall – I shall always remember The CHA CHA CHA as the dance that helped me to control and master the tension felt by all dancers competing for major titles. It is a relaxing dance that has left me with many happy memories.

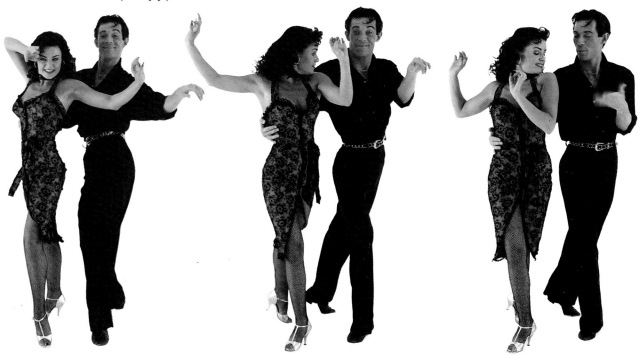

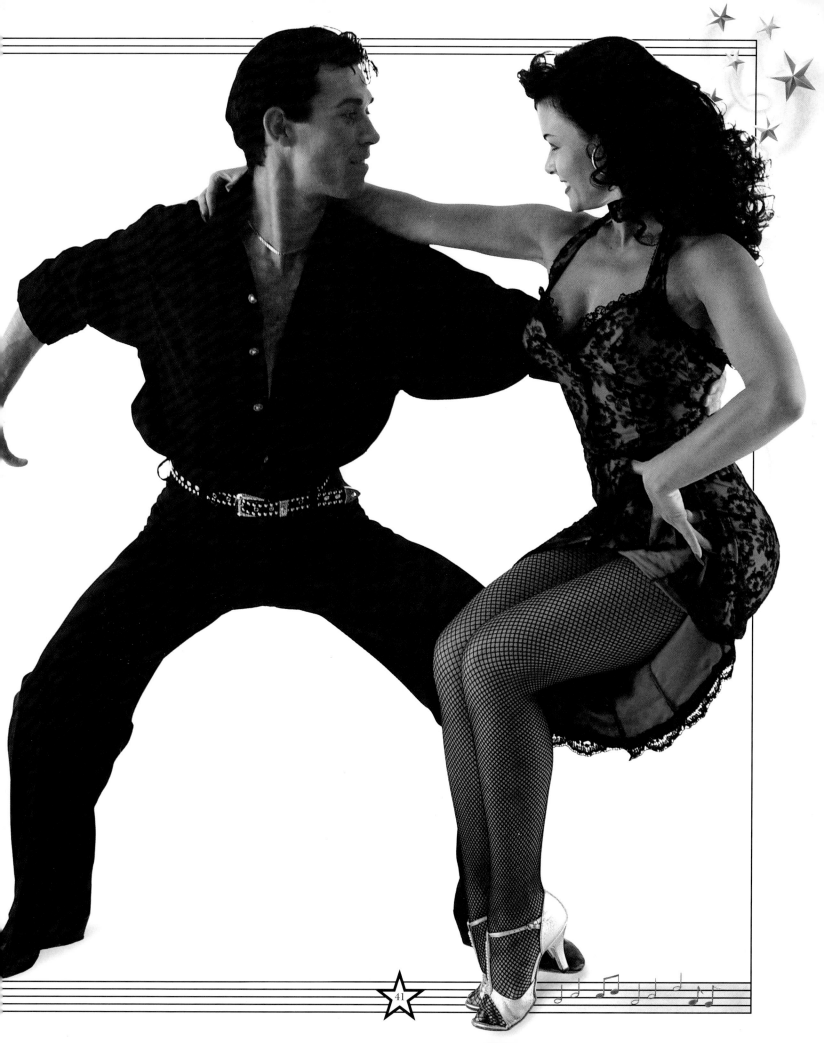

CHA CHA CHA music, which originated in Cuba, has a strong, compelling, easily recognized rhythm that can be counted comfortably as "One, two, three, four and one, two, three, four and one", etc. The beats that occur on the count of "four and one" are accented, and may be spelled out as CHA CHA CHA. Like all Latin American music, CHA CHA CHA music is based on a strong percussion section, which should contain bongos, congas, timbales, and a cowbell. The best tempo for the music is 30 bars per minute. The strongest musical accent occurs on the first beat of each bar.

The CHA CHA CHA consists of some twenty basic figures and innumerable variations developed from these basic figures. However, newcomers to the dance will soon attract the attention of their friends if they can dance well the four basic figures that are illustrated and described on the following pages. Study the photographs and instructions for the correct foot positions and weight distribution; also note carefully the information regarding the Preparatory Step, which must be used to start the dance in correct time with the music. Then all you have to do is turn to Track 7 or 8 on your compact disc, and CHA CHA CHA.

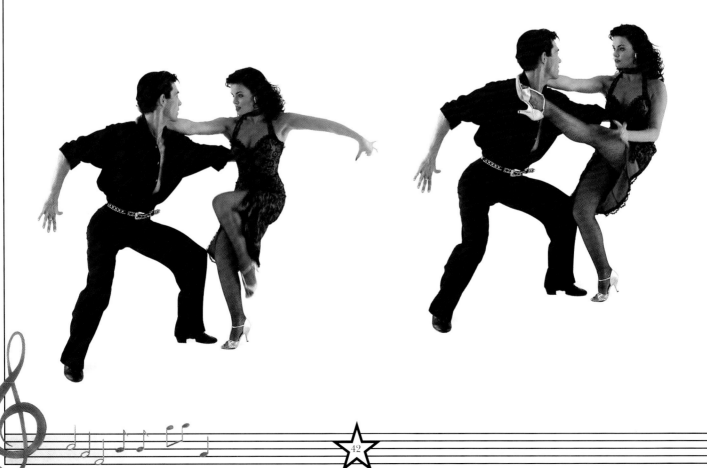

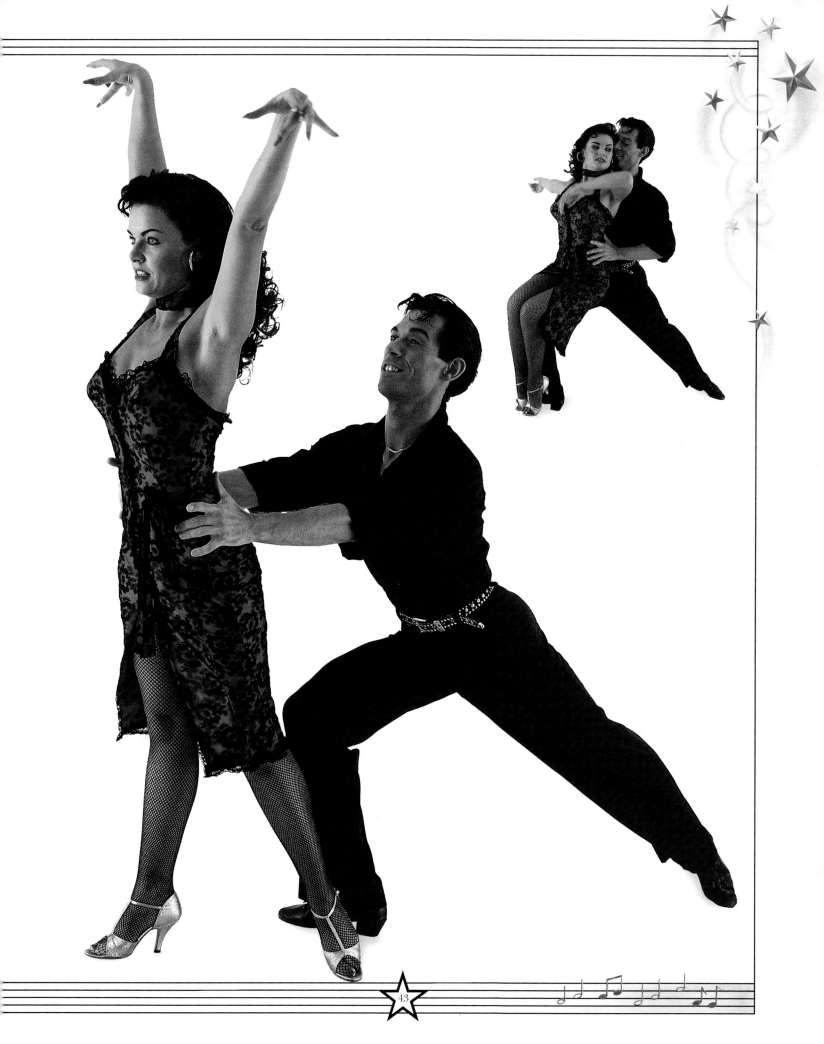

SOLO EXERCISE

STARTING TO MUSIC

This exercise is designed to teach you to make the necessary changes of weight from one foot to the other in time with the music. Steps 3, 4, 5 and steps 8, 9, 10 will coincide with the beats "FOUR AND ONE" of the music – these are the beats that give the dance its name, CHA CHA CHA.

To start this SOLO EXERCISE to music, count "ONE, TWO, THREE, FOUR AND ONE" in time with any bar of the music. Start by taking a Preparatory Step on any count "ONE" of the music.

MAN

Begin with feet together, weight on LF, facing in any direction, arms held slightly foward in a comfortable position. On count "ONE", take a Preparatory Step to side with RF. Dance steps 1 to 10 then repeat *ad lib* from step 1.

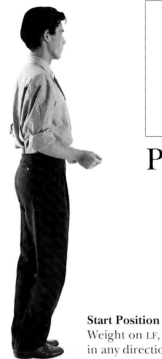

Start Position
Weight on LF, facing in any direction

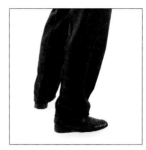

COUNT "ONE"

PREPARATORY STEP
RF to side

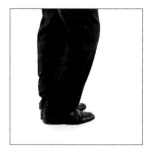

COUNT "TWO"

1 LF closed to RF

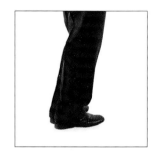

COUNT "TWO"

6 RF closed to LF

WOMAN

Begin with feet together, weight on RF, facing in any direction, arms held slightly foward in a comfortable position. On count "ONE", take a Preparatory Step to side with LF. Dance steps 1 to 10, then repeat *ad lib* from step 1.

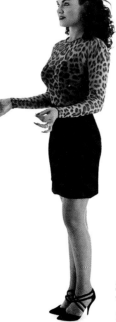

Start Position
Weight on RF, facing in any direction

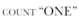
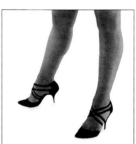

COUNT "ONE"

PREPARATORY STEP
LF to side

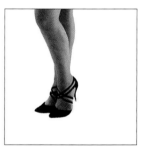

COUNT "TWO"

1 RF closed to LF

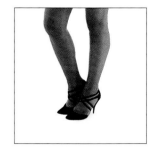

COUNT "TWO"

6 LF closed to RF

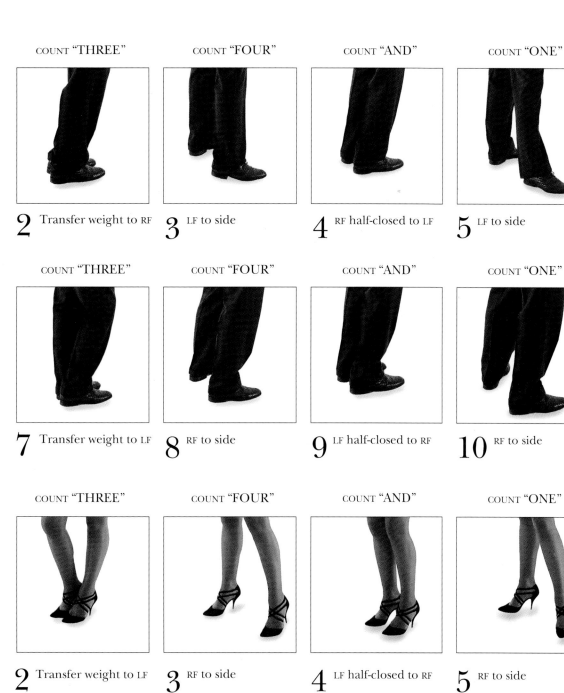

COUNT "THREE"   COUNT "FOUR"   COUNT "AND"   COUNT "ONE"

2 Transfer weight to RF   **3** LF to side   **4** RF half-closed to LF   **5** LF to side

COUNT "THREE"   COUNT "FOUR"   COUNT "AND"   COUNT "ONE"

Repeat *ad lib* from step 1

7 Transfer weight to LF   **8** RF to side   **9** LF half-closed to RF   **10** RF to side

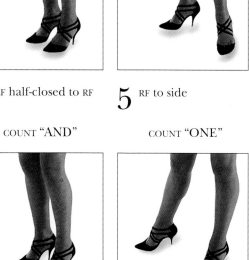

COUNT "THREE"   COUNT "FOUR"   COUNT "AND"   COUNT "ONE"

2 Transfer weight to LF   **3** RF to side   **4** LF half-closed to RF   **5** RF to side

COUNT "THREE"   COUNT "FOUR"   COUNT "AND"   COUNT "ONE"

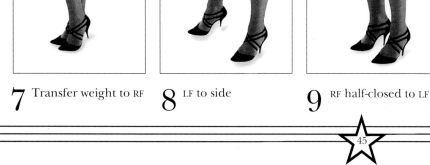

Repeat *ad lib* from step 1

7 Transfer weight to RF   **8** LF to side   **9** RF half-closed to LF   **10** LF to side

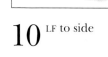

CLOSE HOLD

The CLOSE HOLD for The CHA CHA CHA, as with other Latin dances, is not the same as for the Modern dances. The major difference is that there is no body contact between the two partners and a more relaxed stance is used.

MAN   **WOMAN**

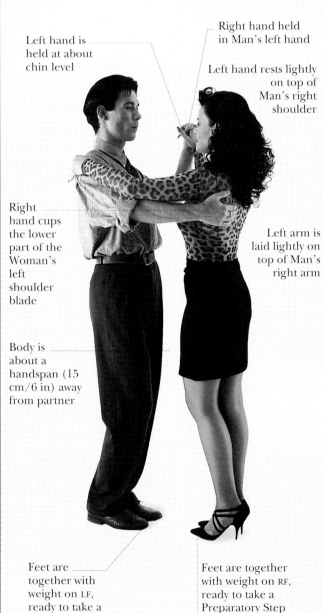

Left hand is held at about chin level

Right hand held in Man's left hand

Left hand rests lightly on top of Man's right shoulder

Right hand cups the lower part of the Woman's left shoulder blade

Left arm is laid lightly on top of Man's right arm

Body is about a handspan (15 cm/6 in) away from partner

Feet are together with weight on LF, ready to take a Preparatory Step on the RF

Feet are together with weight on RF, ready to take a Preparatory Step on the LF

THE CLOSE BASIC   Begin in CLOSE HOLD (see Box, left), with weight on LF (Woman RF), facing in any direction.

COUNT "ONE"   COUNT "TWO"

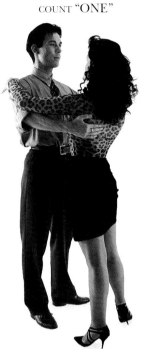

PREPARATORY STEP
M ~ RF to side and slightly forward
W ~ LF to side and slightly back

1 **M** ~ LF forward, toe turned out
W ~ RF back

COUNT "TWO"

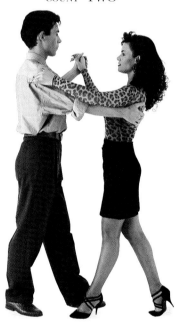

6 **M** ~ RF back
W ~ LF forward, toe turned out

* Repeat *ad lib* from step 1, or continue with THE CLOSE BASIC WITH UNDER ARM TURN TO RIGHT

COUNT "THREE"   COUNT "FOUR"   COUNT "AND"   COUNT "ONE"

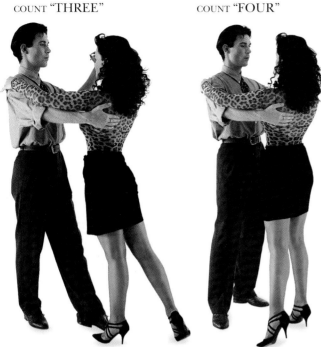 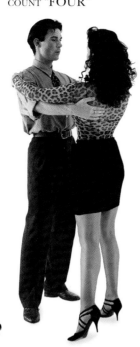 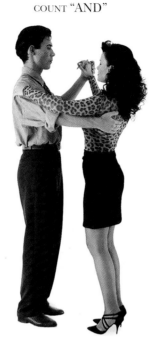 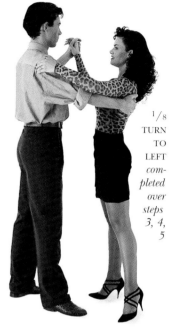

¹/₈ TURN TO LEFT *completed over steps 3, 4, 5*

2 **M** ~ Transfer weight to RF
W ~ Transfer weight to LF

3 **M** ~ LF to side and slightly back
W ~ RF to side and slightly forward

4 **M** ~ RF half-closed to LF
W ~ LF half-closed to RF

5 **M** ~ LF to side and slightly back
W ~ RF to side and slightly forward

COUNT "THREE"   COUNT "FOUR"   COUNT "AND"   COUNT "ONE"

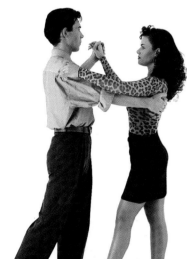 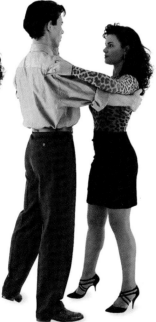 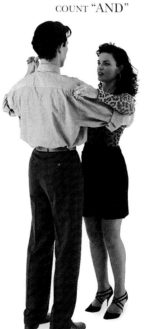 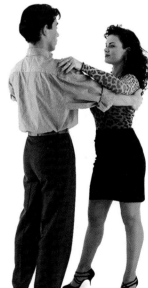

¹/₈ TURN TO LEFT *completed over steps 8, 9, 10*

7 **M** ~ Transfer weight to LF
W ~ Transfer weight to RF

8 **M** ~ RF to side and slightly forward
W ~ LF to side and slightly back

9 **M** ~ LF half-closed to RF
W ~ RF half-closed to LF

10 **M** ~ RF to side and slightly forward *
W ~ LF to side and slightly back *

THE CLOSE BASIC WITH UNDER ARM TURN TO RIGHT

COUNT "TWO" COUNT "THREE"

Begin in CLOSE HOLD, weight on LF (Woman RF), facing in any direction, after dancing steps 1 to 5 of THE CLOSE BASIC.

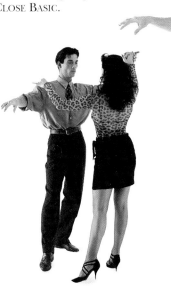
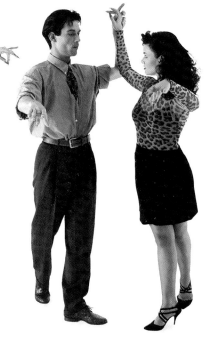

1-5 Dance steps 1 to 5 of THE CLOSE BASIC, releasing hold with RIGHT hand on step 5

6 **M** ~ RF back, raising LEFT arm
W ~ LF forward, turning to RIGHT under Man's upraised LEFT arm to finish LF back

7 **M** ~ Transfer weight to LF
W ~ Transfer weight to RF

THE CLOSE BASIC FINISHED IN OPEN CPP

COUNT "TWO" COUNT "THREE"

Begin in CLOSE HOLD, weight on LF (Woman RF), facing in any direction, after dancing steps 1 to 5 of THE CLOSE BASIC.

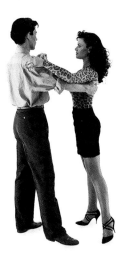
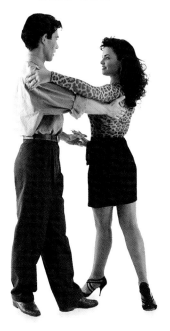
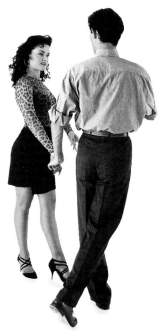

1-5 Dance steps 1 to 5 of THE CLOSE BASIC

6 **M** ~ RF back, lowering LEFT arm, Woman outside
W ~ LF forward, outside Man

7 **M** ~ Transfer weight to LF, releasing hold with RIGHT hand
W ~ RF forward, turning to LEFT

COUNT "FOUR"

COUNT "AND"

COUNT "ONE"

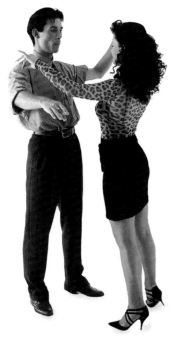

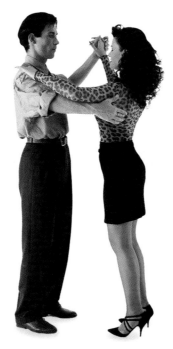

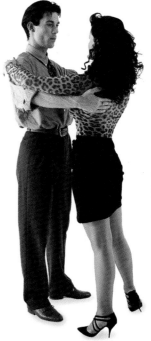

Continue with
THE CLOSE
BASIC FINISHED
IN OPEN CPP

ONE TURN TO
RIGHT *completed*
by *Woman over
steps 6, 7, 8,
9, 10*

8 **M** ~ RF to side
W ~ LF to side

9 **M** ~ LF half-closed to RF
W ~ RF half-closed to LF

10 **M** ~ RF to side and slightly forward,
achieving CLOSE HOLD
W ~ LF to side and slightly back

COUNT "FOUR"

COUNT "AND"

COUNT "ONE"

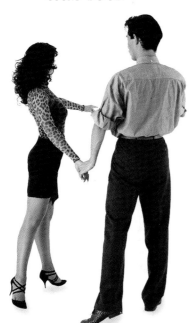

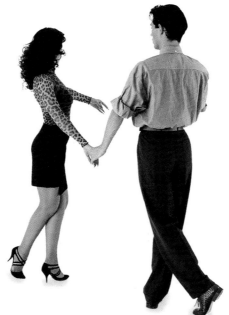

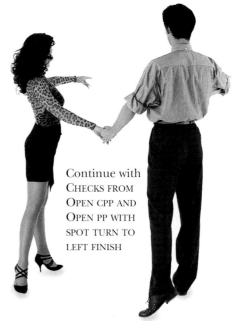

Continue with
CHECKS FROM
OPEN CPP AND
OPEN PP WITH
SPOT TURN TO
LEFT FINISH

8 **M** ~ RF forward
W ~ LF forward

9 **M** ~ LF crossed behind RF
W ~ RF crossed behind LF

10 **M** ~ RF to side in OPEN CPP
W ~ LF to side in OPEN CPP

CHECKS FROM OPEN CPP AND OPEN PP WITH SPOT TURN TO LEFT FINISH

Begin in OPEN CPP with weight on RF (Woman LF), facing in any direction, after dancing THE CLOSE BASIC FINISHED IN OPEN CPP.

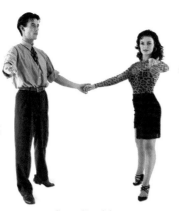

Start Position
Weight on RF (Woman LF) in OPEN CPP

COUNT "TWO"

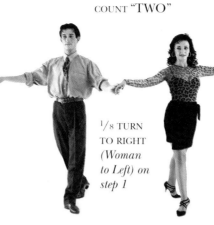

¹/₈ TURN TO RIGHT *(Woman to Left) on step 1*

1 **M** ~ LF forward, toe turned out
W ~ RF forward, toe turned out

COUNT "THREE"

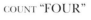

2 **M** ~ Transfer weight to RF
W ~ Transfer weight to LF

COUNT "THREE"

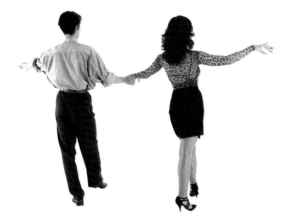

7 **M** ~ Transfer weight to LF
W ~ Transfer weight to RF

COUNT "FOUR"

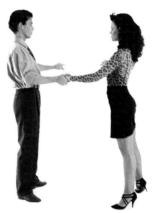

8 **M** ~ RF to side
W ~ LF to side

COUNT "AND"

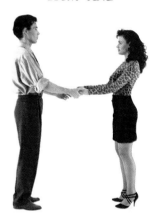

9 **M** ~ LF half-closed to RF, releasing hold with RIGHT hand and achieving LEFT-TO-RIGHT hand hold
W ~ RF half-closed to LF

COUNT "FOUR"

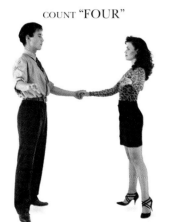

13 **M** ~ LF to side
W ~ RF to side

COUNT "AND"

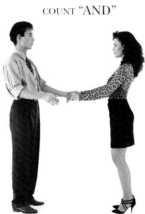

14 **M** ~ RF half-closed to LF, releasing hold with LEFT hand
W ~ LF half-closed to RF

COUNT "ONE"

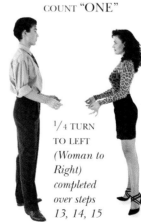

¹/₄ TURN TO LEFT *(Woman to Right) completed over steps 13, 14, 15*

15 **M** ~ LF to side
W ~ RF to side

COUNT "TWO"

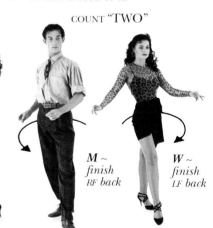

M ~ finish RF back

W ~ finish LF back

16 **M** ~ RF forward across LF, turning to LEFT
W ~ LF forward across RF, turning to RIGHT

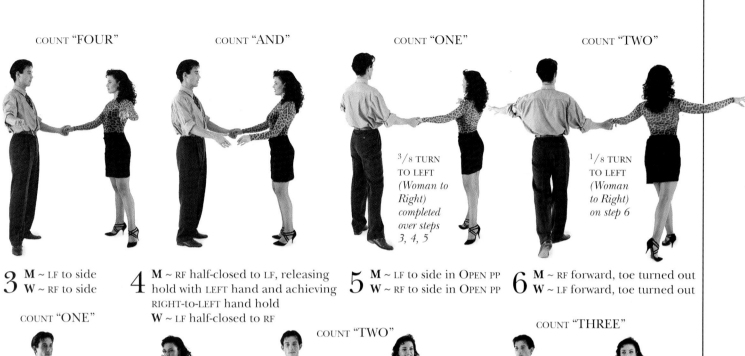

COUNT "FOUR"

COUNT "AND"

COUNT "ONE"

3/8 TURN TO LEFT (Woman to Right) completed over steps 3, 4, 5

COUNT "TWO"

1/8 TURN TO LEFT (Woman to Right) on step 6

3 M ~ LF to side
W ~ RF to side

4 M ~ RF half-closed to LF, releasing hold with LEFT hand and achieving RIGHT-to-LEFT hand hold
W ~ LF half-closed to RF

5 M ~ LF to side in OPEN PP
W ~ RF to side in OPEN PP

6 M ~ RF forward, toe turned out
W ~ LF forward, toe turned out

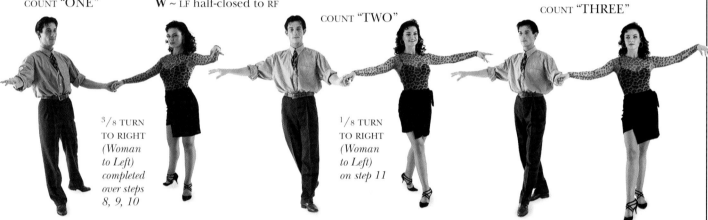

COUNT "ONE"

3/8 TURN TO RIGHT (Woman to Left) completed over steps 8, 9, 10

COUNT "TWO"

1/8 TURN TO RIGHT (Woman to Left) on step 11

COUNT "THREE"

10 M ~ RF to side in OPEN CPP
W ~ LF to side in OPEN CPP

11 M ~ LF forward, toe turned out
W ~ RF forward, toe turned out

12 M ~ Transfer weight to RF
W ~ Transfer weight to LF

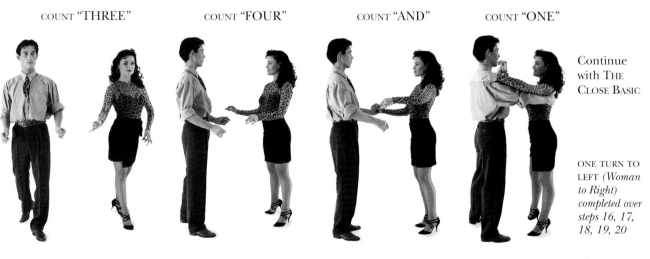

COUNT "THREE"

COUNT "FOUR"

COUNT "AND"

COUNT "ONE"

Continue with THE CLOSE BASIC

ONE TURN TO LEFT *(Woman to Right) completed over steps 16, 17, 18, 19, 20*

17 M ~ Transfer weight to LF
W ~ Transfer weight to RF

18 M ~ RF to side
W ~ LF to side

19 M ~ LF half-closed to RF
W ~ RF half-closed to LF

20 M ~ RF to side; achieve CLOSE HOLD
W ~ LF to side; achieve CLOSE HOLD

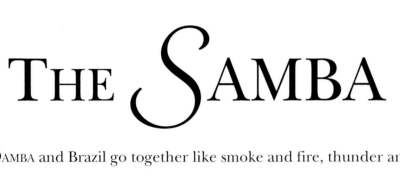

The Samba

Samba and Brazil go together like smoke and fire, thunder and lightning, and night and day. Samba is an integral part of Brazilian culture – it is the music and dance of the people by the people.

Carnival and Samba is another word combination that typifies the mood this music fires in the hearts of the people of Brazil.

Each year, for five nights and five days in February, the workaday life of Rio de Janeiro comes to a standstill – it's Carnival time... a never-ending procession of extravagantly decorated floats, each with its own group of musicians and dancers performing to Samba music that has been especially written for the occasion. The floats weave a bright, colourful, non-stop pattern through the city streets.

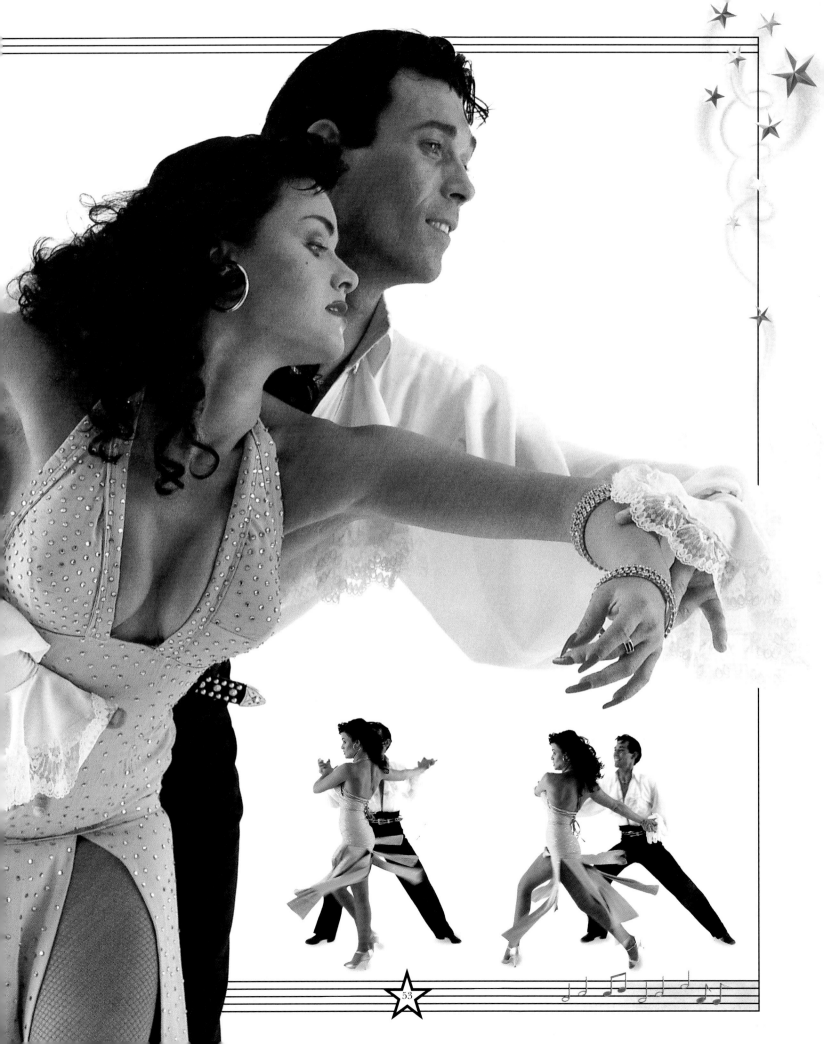

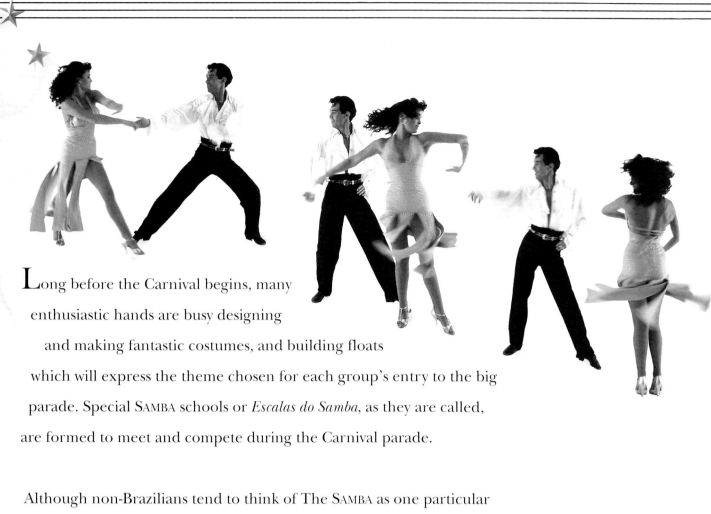

Long before the Carnival begins, many enthusiastic hands are busy designing and making fantastic costumes, and building floats which will express the theme chosen for each group's entry to the big parade. Special SAMBA schools or *Escalas do Samba,* as they are called, are formed to meet and compete during the Carnival parade.

Although non-Brazilians tend to think of The SAMBA as one particular dance, it is not. There are many different versions of The SAMBA – each with a different rhythm, tempo, and mood – resulting in many different dances. The dance the West knows as The SAMBA is just one of these many exciting and thrilling rhythms.

To capture the character of this SAMBA, dancers should adopt a flirtatious and exuberant carnival mood.

Many of the figures used in SAMBA require a particular tilting pelvic action. This is somewhat difficult to learn, but without it, the figures that require it will not look rhythmic or authentic.

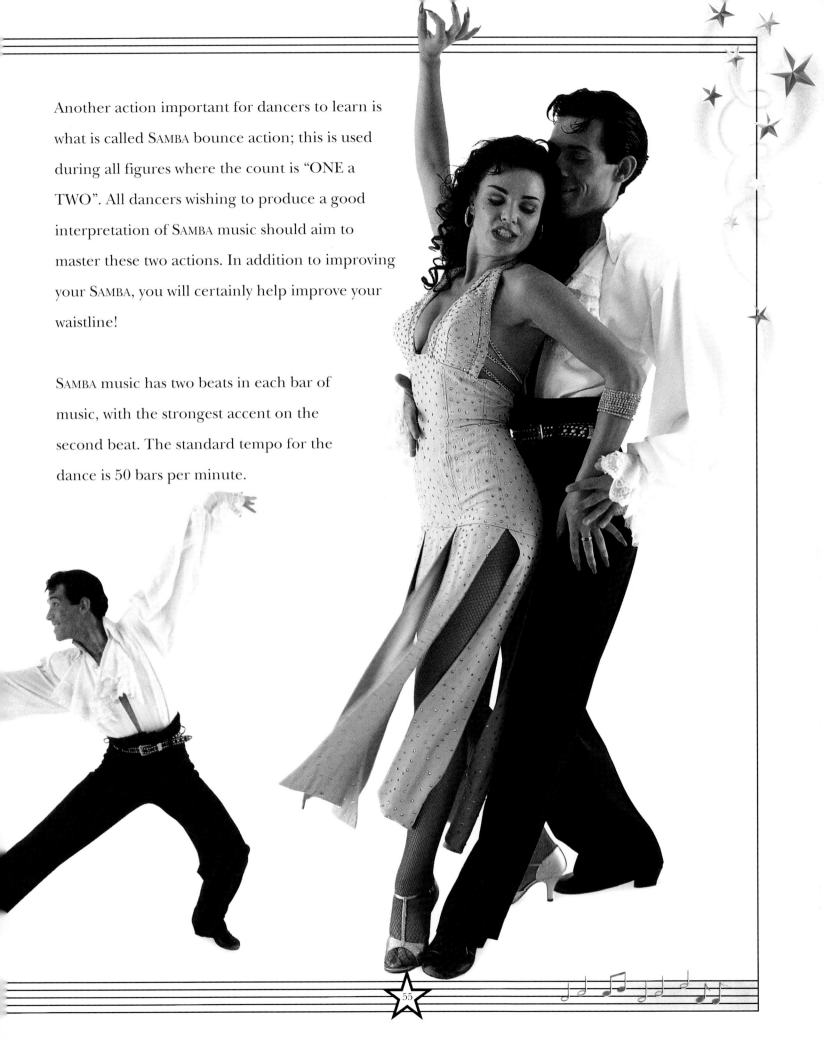

Another action important for dancers to learn is what is called SAMBA bounce action; this is used during all figures where the count is "ONE a TWO". All dancers wishing to produce a good interpretation of SAMBA music should aim to master these two actions. In addition to improving your SAMBA, you will certainly help improve your waistline!

SAMBA music has two beats in each bar of music, with the strongest accent on the second beat. The standard tempo for the dance is 50 bars per minute.

SOLO EXERCISE

STARTING TO MUSIC

If you listen to SAMBA music you will hear three sounds like "gooon...ga...goooon" repeated in each bar of music. All the figures described in this book are danced to these three sounds. When dancing to this rhythm, three steps are used – one for each sound, therefore, "gooon...ga... goooon" becomes a movement of three steps with the timing of "ONE a TWO".

To start the SOLO EXERCISE to music, first count "ONE a TWO" in time with the music until you can clearly hear these three sounds. Count "ONE a TWO" in unison with these sounds. Take step 1 of the exercise on any count of "ONE".

The method described above should be used whenever you start to dance The SAMBA, until it becomes a muscular memory.

SAMBA BOUNCE ACTION

In figures that have the timing "ONE a TWO", each group of three steps involves a flexing of the knees. Begin with the knees compressed. Take the first step using a slight push-off from the standing foot during which the knees will tend to straighten. After the moving foot arrives in position, the knee will soften as the weight is collected onto this foot.

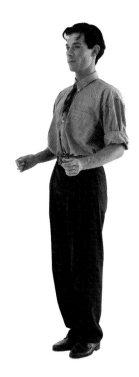

Start position
Weight on RF,
facing in any
direction

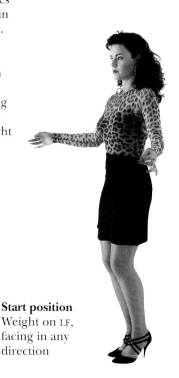

Start position
Weight on LF,
facing in any
direction

MAN

Begin with feet together, weight on RF, both knees compressed, facing in any direction. Use SAMBA bounce action throughout (see text, left). Take the first step on the first beat of any bar of music. Repeat SOLO EXERCISE *ad lib.*

COUNT "ONE"   COUNT "a"

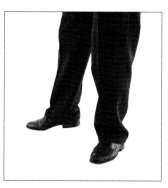   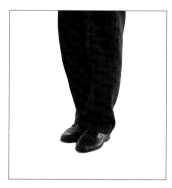

1 LF to side   **2** RF, with part weight, closed to LF

WOMAN

Begin with feet together, weight on LF, both knees compressed, facing in any direction. Use SAMBA bounce action throughout (see text, left). Take the first step on the first beat of any bar of music. Repeat SOLO EXERCISE *ad lib.*

COUNT "ONE"   COUNT "a"

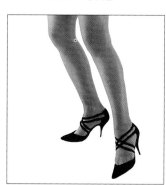   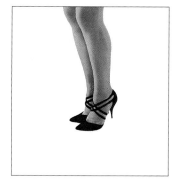

1 RF to side   **2** LF, with part weight, closed to RF

COUNT "TWO"

COUNT "ONE"

COUNT "a"

COUNT "TWO"

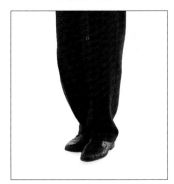

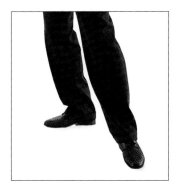

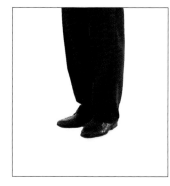

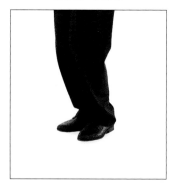

3 Transfer full weight to LF

4 RF to side

5 LF, with part weight, closed to RF

6 Transfer full weight to RF

COUNT "TWO"

COUNT "ONE"

COUNT "a"

COUNT "TWO"

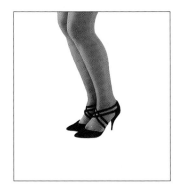

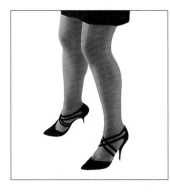

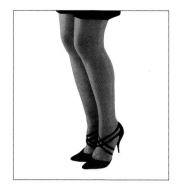

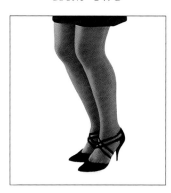

3 Transfer full weight to RF

4 LF to side

5 RF, with part weight, closed to LF

6 Transfer full weight to LF

CLOSE HOLD

In the CLOSE HOLD for The SAMBA, there is no body contact between partners and a more relaxed stance is used.

MAN

WOMAN

Right hand held in partner's left hand

Left hand is held at chin level

Left hand rests lightly on top of Man's right shoulder

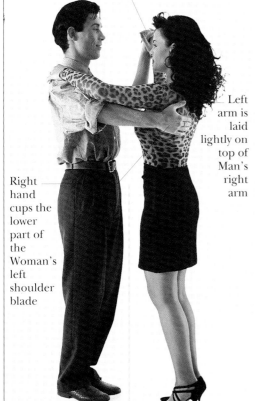

Left arm is laid lightly on top of Man's right arm

Right hand cups the lower part of the Woman's left shoulder blade

Feet are together with weight on LF or RF, depending on figure to be danced

Body is about a handspan (15 cm/ 6 in) away from partner

Feet are together with weight on RF or LF (decided by Man)

ALIGNMENT

Because the SAMBA is a moving dance during which there is progression around the dance floor in an anti-clockwise direction, each figure has a definite start and finish position in relation to the room.

THE NATURAL BASIC

COUNT "ONE"

COUNT "a"

Begin in CLOSE HOLD (see Box, left), with weight on LF (Woman RF), facing LOD. Keep all steps small; don't try to travel.

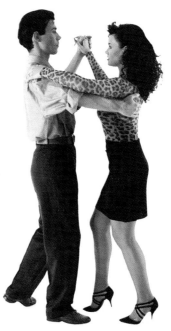
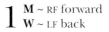
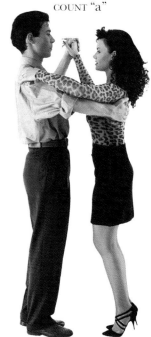

1 M ~ RF forward
W ~ LF back

2 M ~ LF, with part weight, closed to RF
W ~ RF, with part weight, closed to LF

THE PROGRESSIVE BASIC

COUNT "ONE"

COUNT "a"

Begin in CLOSE HOLD (see Box, left), weight on LF (Woman RF), facing LOD. Keep all steps small; don't try to travel.

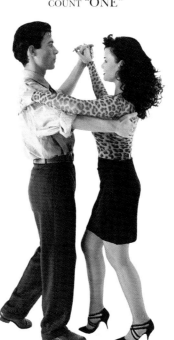
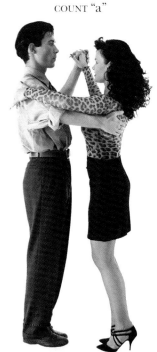

1 M ~ RF forward
W ~ LF back

2 M ~ LF, with part weight, closed to RF
W ~ RF, with part weight, closed to LF

* Repeat *ad lib* from step 1, or continue with THE PROGRESSIVE BASIC

COUNT "TWO"   COUNT "ONE"   COUNT "a"   COUNT "TWO"

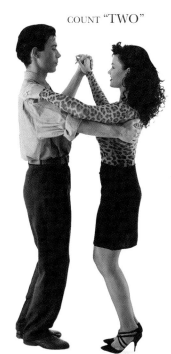 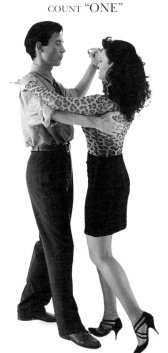 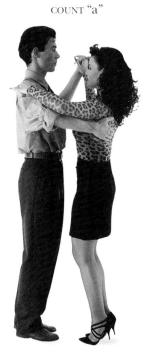 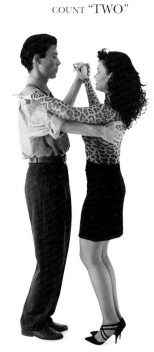

3 **M** ~ Transfer full weight to RF
W ~Transfer full weight to LF

4 **M** ~ LF back
W ~ RF forward

5 **M** ~ RF, with part weight, closed to LF
W ~ LF, with part weight, closed to RF

6 **M** ~ Transfer full weight to LF *
W ~Transfer full weight to RF *

** Repeat *ad lib* from step 1, or continue with THE NATURAL BASIC

COUNT "TWO"   COUNT "ONE"   COUNT "a"   COUNT "TWO"

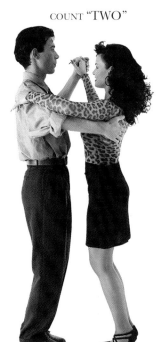 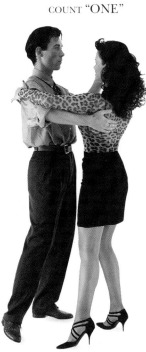 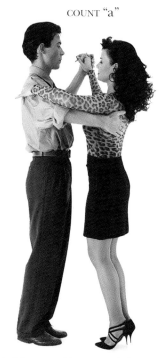 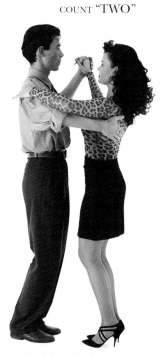

3 **M** ~ Transfer full weight to RF
W ~ Transfer full weight to LF

4 **M** ~ LF to side
W ~ RF to side

5 **M** ~ RF, with part weight, closed to LF
W ~ LF, with part weight, closed to RF

6 **M** ~ Transfer full weight to LF **
W ~ Transfer full weight to RF **

WHISK TO LEFT

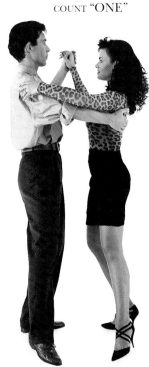

COUNT "ONE"

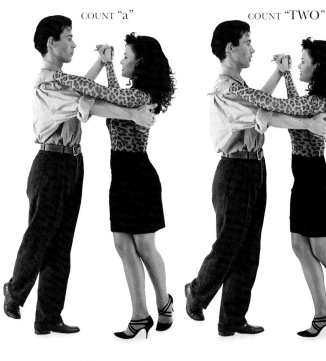

COUNT "a"   COUNT "TWO"

Begin in CLOSE HOLD (see Box, p.58), with weight on RF (Woman LF), facing wall.

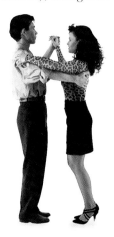

Continue with WHISK TO RIGHT

Start Position
Weight on RF (Woman LF), facing wall

1 **M** ~ LF to side
W ~ RF to side

2 **M** ~ RF, with part weight, crossed behind LF
W ~ LF, with part weight, crossed behind RF

3 **M** ~ Transfer full weight to LF
W ~ Transfer full weight to RF

UNDER ARM TURN TO RIGHT

Begin in CLOSE HOLD, with weight on RF (Woman LF), facing wall, having danced WHISK TO RIGHT.

COUNT "ONE"   COUNT "a"   COUNT "TWO"

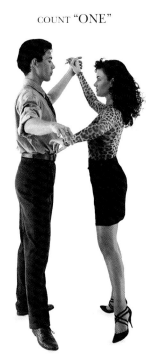

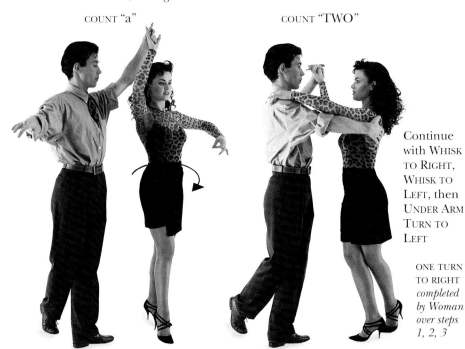

Continue with WHISK TO RIGHT, WHISK TO LEFT, then UNDER ARM TURN TO LEFT

ONE TURN TO RIGHT *completed by Woman over steps 1, 2, 3*

1 **M** ~ LF to side, raising LEFT arm and releasing RIGHT hand
W ~ RF forward starting to turn to RIGHT

2 **M** ~ RF, with part weight, crossed behind LF
W ~ Turning strongly to RIGHT, LF, with part weight, back

3 **M** ~ Transfer full weight to LF, achieving CLOSE HOLD
W ~ Transfer full weight to RF still turning to RIGHT. Finish with RF crossed in front of LF

WHISK TO RIGHT

Begin in CLOSE HOLD, with weight on LF (Woman RF), facing wall, having danced WHISK TO LEFT.

COUNT "ONE"   COUNT "a"   COUNT "TWO"

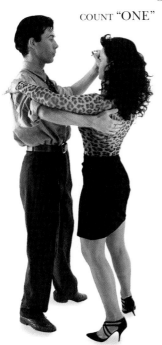 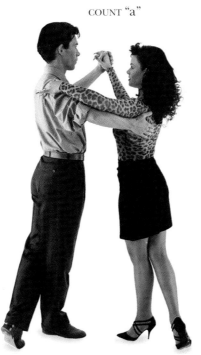 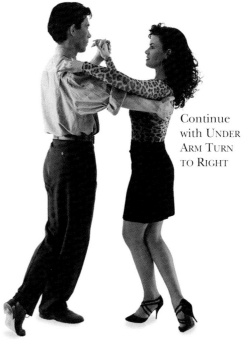

Continue with UNDER ARM TURN TO RIGHT

1 M ~ RF to side
W ~ LF to side

2 M ~ LF, with part weight, crossed behind RF
W ~ RF, with part weight, crossed behind LF

3 M ~ Transfer full weight to RF
W ~ Transfer full weight to LF

UNDER ARM TURN TO LEFT

Begin in CLOSE HOLD, with weight on LF (Woman RF), facing wall, having danced WHISK TO LEFT.

COUNT "ONE"   COUNT "a"   COUNT "TWO"

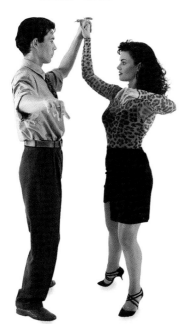 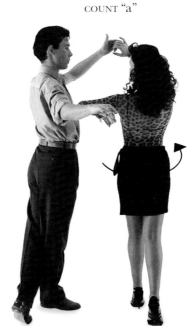 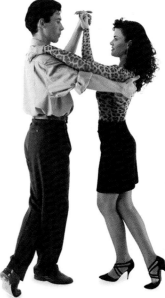

Continue with a WHISK TO LEFT and WHISK TO RIGHT TURNED TO PP

ONE TURN TO LEFT *completed by Woman over steps 1, 2, 3*

1 M ~ RF to side, raising LEFT arm and releasing RIGHT hand
W ~ LF forward starting to turn to LEFT

2 M ~ LF, with part weight, crossed behind RF
W ~ Turning strongly to LEFT, RF, with part weight, back

3 M ~ Transfer full weight to RF, achieving CLOSE HOLD
W ~ Still turning to LEFT, transfer full weight to LF. Finish with LF crossed in front of RF

WHISK TO RIGHT TURNED TO PP

Begin in CLOSE HOLD weight on LF (Woman RF), facing wall, having danced WHISK TO LEFT.

COUNT "ONE"

COUNT "a"

COUNT "TWO"

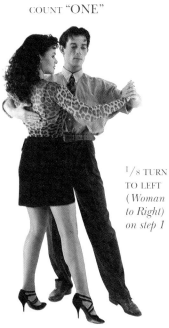

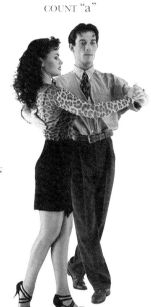

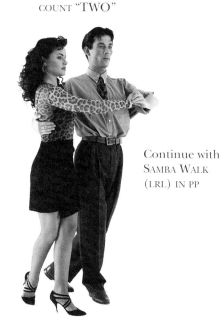

¹/₈ TURN TO LEFT (Woman to Right) on step 1

Continue with SAMBA WALK (LRL) IN PP

1 **M** ~ RF to side, turning to LEFT
W ~ LF to side, turning to RIGHT

2 **M** ~ LF, with part weight, crossed behind RF
W ~ RF, with part weight, crossed behind LF

3 **M** ~ Transfer full weight to RF in PP
W ~ Transfer full weight to LF in PP

SAMBA WALK (RLR) IN PP

Begin in PP, on LOD, weight on LF (Woman RF), having danced SAMBA WALK (LRL) IN PP.

COUNT "ONE"

COUNT "a"

COUNT "TWO"

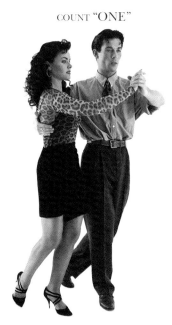

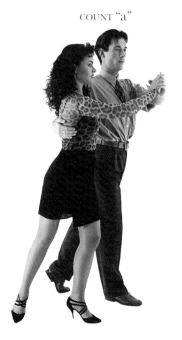

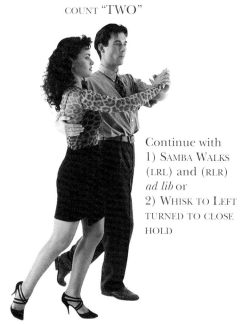

Continue with
1) SAMBA WALKS (LRL) and (RLR) *ad lib* or
2) WHISK TO LEFT TURNED TO CLOSE HOLD

1 **M** ~ RF forward in PP, pelvis tilted forward
W ~ LF forward in PP, pelvis tilted forward

2 **M** ~ LF back with part weight on inside edge of toe, pelvis tilted back
W ~ RF back with part weight on inside edge of toe, pelvis tilted back

3 **M** ~ Slip RF back (approx. 7.5cm/3in) in PP, pelvis normal, full weight on RF
W ~ Slip LF back (approx. 7.5cm/3in) in PP, pelvis normal, full weight on LF

SAMBA WALK (LRL) IN PP

Begin in PP,
on LOD, weight
on RF (Woman
LF), having
danced WHISK
TO RIGHT
TURNED TO PP.

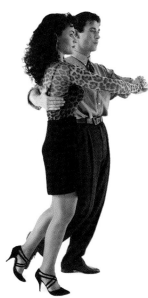

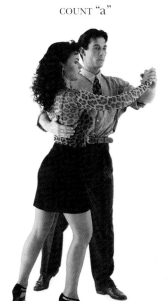

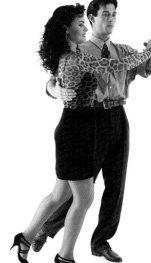

Continue with
SAMBA WALK
(RLR) IN PP

1   **M** ~ LF forward in PP,
pelvis tilted forward
W ~ RF forward in PP,
pelvis tilted forward

2   **M** ~ RF back with part weight on
inside edge of toe, pelvis tilted back
W ~ LF back with part weight on
inside edge of toe, pelvis tilted back

3   **M** ~ Slip LF back (approx 7.5cm/3in) in PP,
pelvis normal; full weight on LF
W ~ Slip RF back (approx 7.5cm/3in) in PP,
pelvis normal; full weight on RF

WHISK TO LEFT TURNED TO CLOSE HOLD

Begin in PP, on
LOD, weight on RF
(Woman LF), having
danced SAMBA WALK
(RLR) IN PP.

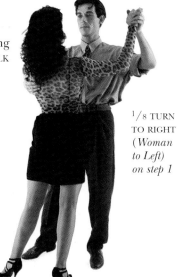

¹/₈ TURN
TO RIGHT
(*Woman
to Left*)
on step 1

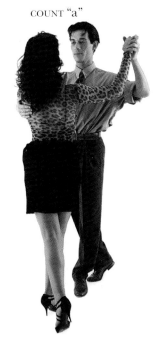

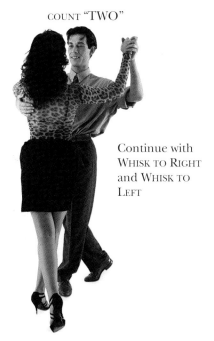

Continue with
WHISK TO RIGHT
and WHISK TO
LEFT

1   **M** ~ LF to side, turning to RIGHT to face
partner in CLOSE HOLD
W ~ RF to side turning to LEFT to face
partner in CLOSE HOLD

2   **M** ~ RF, with part weight, crossed
behind LF
W ~ LF, with part weight, crossed
behind RF

3   **M** ~ Transfer full weight to LF
W ~ Transfer full weight to RF

THE RUMBA

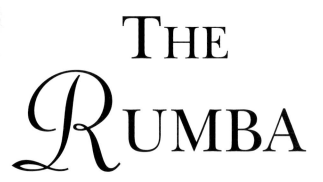

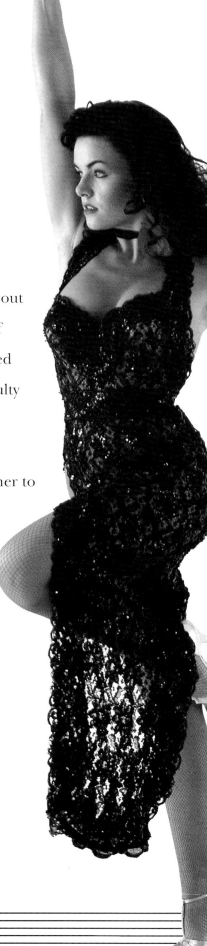

The RUMBA, or more correctly The CUBAN RUMBA, is, without doubt, the most popular dance among the vast majority of Latin dancers. The principles upon which the dance is based are disarmingly simple, but they represent a degree of difficulty that takes many years to perfect.

The RUMBA is a dance that is relatively simple for the beginner to learn; he or she will attain a reasonable degree of success fairly quickly. The same dance, however, is the focus of much time and effort by every top-line competition dancer throughout his or her career. To dance a good RUMBA is the aim of all dedicated Latin dance aficionados.

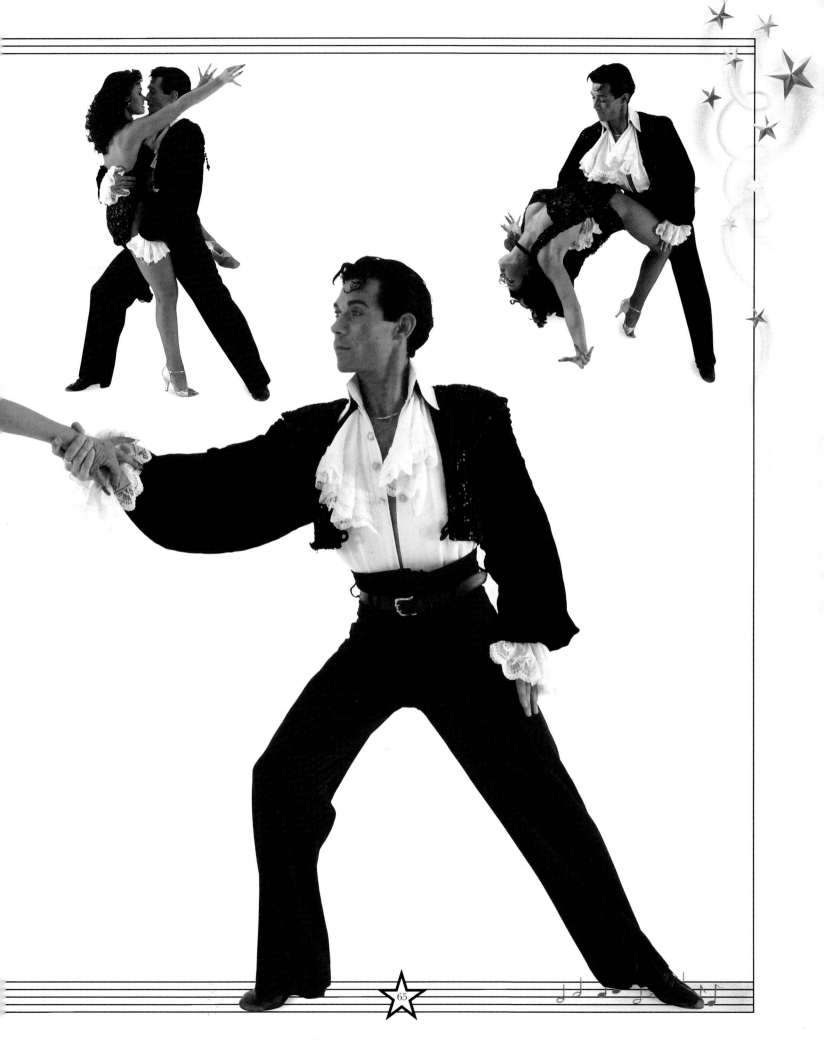

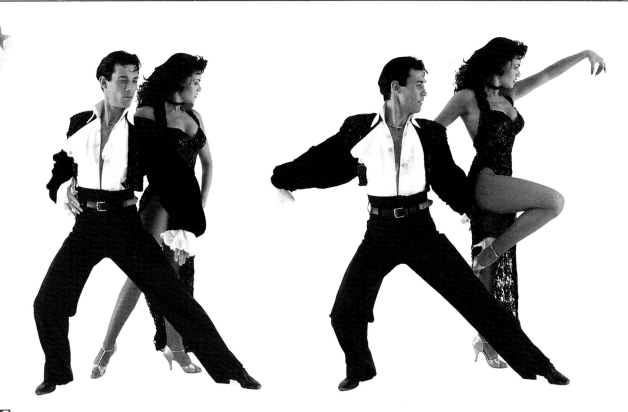

Throughout its long history, The RUMBA has played many roles. It began as a fertility dance during which the dancers mimicked the courtship displays of birds and animals prior to mating. Later versions of The RUMBA humanized these sexual connotations; to the throbbing, insistent beat of the music's erotic rhythm, the woman produced sensuous and inviting movements to attract the attention of the man of her choice.

Much of the choreography used in today's RUMBA retains the age-old story of the woman's attempts to attract and ultimately dominate the man by the use of her feminine charms. During a well-choreographed RUMBA, there will always be an element of tease and run; the man is first lured and then rejected by his partner. The sensuous and erotic invitations by the woman will be answered by the man who expresses his macho image by performing physical feats in an attempt to win her favours.

The five figures described in this section have been chosen to teach you how to dance an authentic rhythmic interpretation of The CUBAN RUMBA – a dance that is considered by top-class dancers to be the classic of all Latin dances.

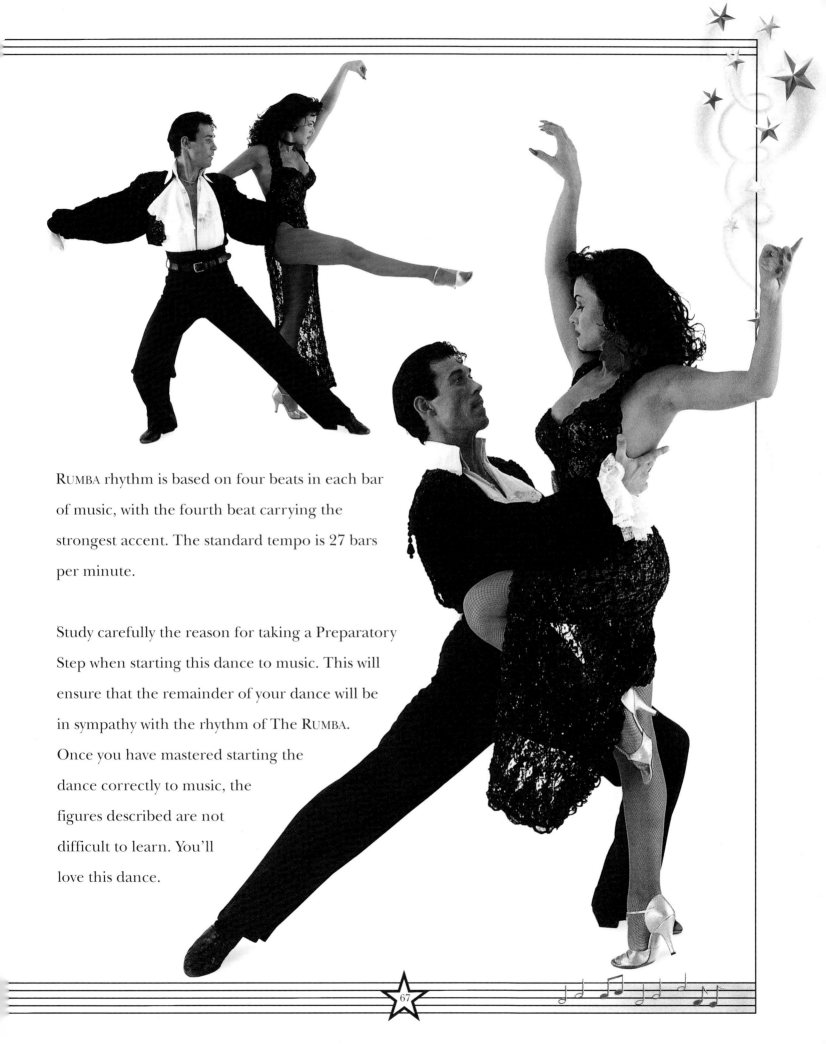

RUMBA rhythm is based on four beats in each bar of music, with the fourth beat carrying the strongest accent. The standard tempo is 27 bars per minute.

Study carefully the reason for taking a Preparatory Step when starting this dance to music. This will ensure that the remainder of your dance will be in sympathy with the rhythm of The RUMBA. Once you have mastered starting the dance correctly to music, the figures described are not difficult to learn. You'll love this dance.

SOLO EXERCISE

This exercise is designed to help you to dance using the authentic interpretation of RUMBA music. It can be danced also with your partner in CLOSE HOLD.

Because Rumba rhythm produces strong accents on beats "FOUR•ONE" of the music, it is necessary for dancers to take a Preparatory Step to the side on this count every time the dance is started to music. Count "ONE, TWO, THREE, FOUR•ONE", etc. in time with the music, then take a Prepatory Step on any count of "FOUR•ONE".

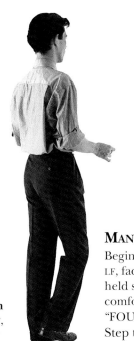

Start Position
Weight on LF, facing in any direction

MAN

Begin with feet together, weight on LF, facing in any direction, arms held slightly forward in a comfortable position. On count "FOUR•ONE", take a Preparatory Step to side with RF. Dance steps 1 to 6 then repeat *ad lib* from step 1.

COUNT "FOUR•ONE"

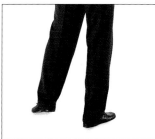

PREPARATORY STEP
RF to side

COUNT "TWO"

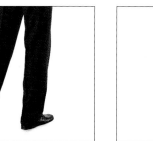

1 LF closed to RF

COUNT "TWO"

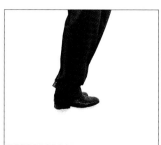

4 RF closed to LF

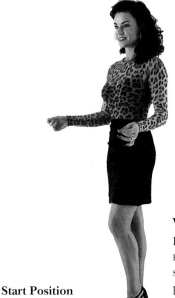

Start Position
Weight on RF, facing in any direction

WOMAN

Begin with feet together, weight on RF, facing in any direction, arms held slightly forward in a comfortable position. On count "FOUR•ONE", take a Preparatory Step to side with LF. Dance steps 1 to 6 then repeat *ad lib* from step 1.

COUNT "FOUR•ONE"

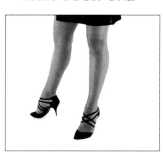

PREPARATORY STEP
LF to side

COUNT "TWO"

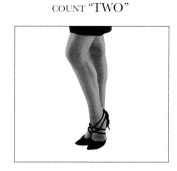

1 RF closed to LF

COUNT "TWO"

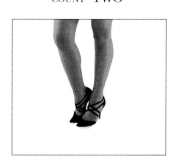

4 LF closed to RF

COUNT "THREE"

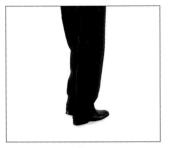

2 Transfer weight to RF

COUNT "FOUR•ONE"

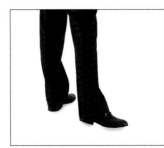

3 LF to side

COUNT "THREE"

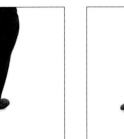

5 Transfer weight to LF

COUNT "FOUR•ONE"

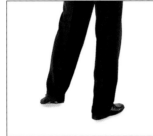

6 RF to side
Repeat *ad lib* from step 1

COUNT "THREE"

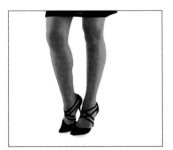

2 Transfer weight to LF

COUNT "FOUR•ONE"

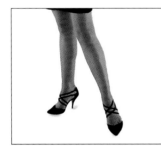

3 RF to side

COUNT "THREE"

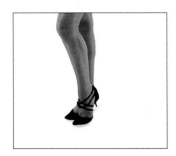

5 Transfer weight to RF

COUNT "FOUR•ONE"

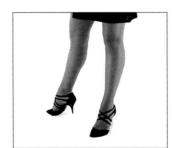

6 LF to side
Repeat *ad lib* from step 1

DANCING TO MUSIC

To dance in sympathy with the rhythm of RUMBA music, it is important that the forward and backward steps (break) used in THE CLOSE BASIC are taken on the second beat of any bar of music. The correct way to achieve this is to begin with weight on the LF (Woman RF) and then take a step RF to side and slightly forward (Woman LF to side and slightly back) on the count of "FOUR•ONE".

CLOSE HOLD

MAN

The left hand is held at about chin level

Right hand cups the lower part of the Woman's left shoulder blade

The body is about a handspan (15 cm/ 6 in) away from partner

Feet together with weight on LF, ready to take a Preparatory Step on the RF

WOMAN

Right hand held in partner's left hand

The left arm is laid lightly on top of the Man's right arm

Left hand rests lightly on top of Man's right shoulder

Feet together with weight on RF, ready to take a Preparatory Step on the LF

ALIGNMENT

Because the Rumba is not a moving dance (i.e. the figures do not move around the dance floor), figures in this dance can be started and finished facing in any direction.

THE CLOSE BASIC

Begin in CLOSE HOLD (see Box, p.69), with weight on LF (Woman RF), facing in any direction.

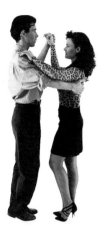

Start Position
Weight on LF
(Woman RF)

COUNT "FOUR•ONE"

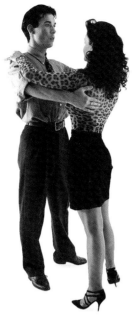

PREPARATORY STEP
M ~ RF to side and slightly forward
W ~ LF to side and slightly back

COUNT "TWO"

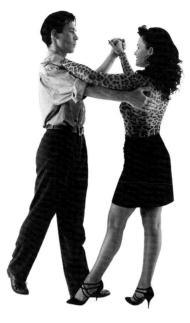

1 **M** ~ LF forward, toe turned out
W ~ RF back

COUNT "THREE"

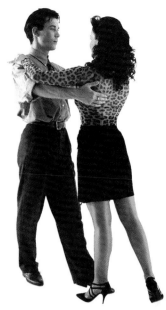

2 **M** ~ Transfer weight to RF
W ~ Transfer weight to LF

THE CLOSE BASIC WITH UNDER ARM TURN TO RIGHT

Begin in CLOSE HOLD, weight on LF (Woman RF), facing in any direction, having danced steps 1 to 3 of THE CLOSE BASIC.

* Continue with THE CLOSE BASIC FINISHED IN OPEN CPP

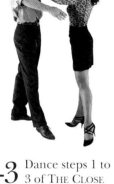

COUNT "TWO"

COUNT "THREE"

COUNT "FOUR•ONE"

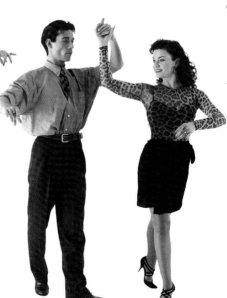

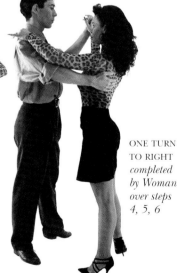

ONE TURN TO RIGHT *completed by Woman over steps 4, 5, 6*

1-3 Dance steps 1 to 3 of THE CLOSE BASIC, releasing hold with RIGHT hand on step 3

4 **M** ~ RF back, raising LEFT arm
W ~ LF forward, turning strongly to RIGHT, under Man's upraised LEFT arm, to finish LF back

5 **M** ~ Transfer weight to LF
W ~ Transfer weight to RF

6 **M** ~ RF to side and slightly forward, regaining CLOSE HOLD *
W ~ LF to side and slightly back *

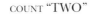

* Repeat *ad lib*, or continue with THE CLOSE BASIC WITH UNDER ARM TURN TO RIGHT

COUNT "FOUR•ONE"   COUNT "TWO"   COUNT "THREE"   COUNT "FOUR•ONE"

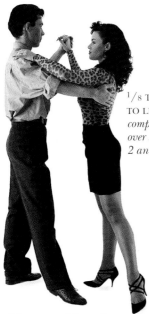 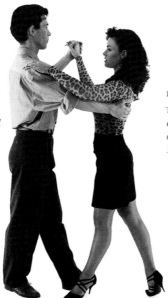 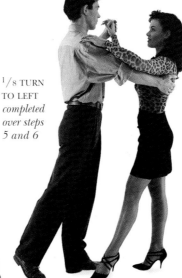 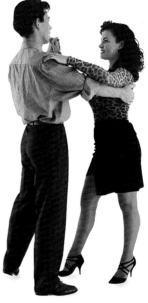

1/8 TURN TO LEFT completed over steps 2 and 3

1/8 TURN TO LEFT completed over steps 5 and 6

3 **M** ~ LF to side and slightly back
W ~ RF to side and slightly forward

4 **M** ~ RF back
W ~ LF forward, toe turned out

5 **M** ~ Transfer weight to LF
W ~ Transfer weight to RF

6 **M** ~ RF to side and slightly forward *
W ~ LF to side and slightly back *

THE CLOSE BASIC FINISHED IN OPEN CPP

** Continue with CHECKS FROM OPEN CPP AND OPEN PP WITH SPOT TURN TO LEFT FINISH

Begin in CLOSE HOLD, weight on LF (Woman RF), facing in any direction, having danced steps 1 to 3 of THE CLOSE BASIC.

COUNT "TWO"   COUNT "THREE"   COUNT "FOUR•ONE"

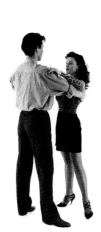 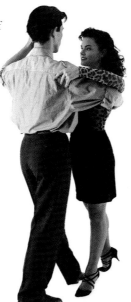 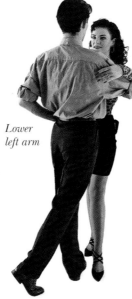 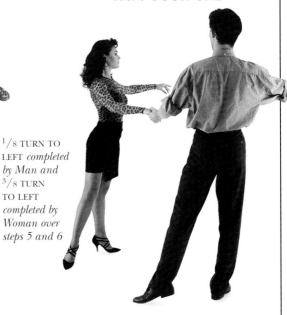

Lower left arm

1/8 TURN TO LEFT completed by Man and 3/8 TURN TO LEFT completed by Woman over steps 5 and 6

1-3 Dance steps 1 to 3 of THE CLOSE BASIC

4 **M** ~ RF back
W ~ LF forward, toward Man

5 **M** ~ Transfer weight to LF
W ~ RF forward (small step), turning to LEFT

6 **M** ~ RF to side in OPEN CPP **
W ~ LF to side in OPEN CPP **

CHECKS FROM OPEN CPP AND OPEN PP WITH SPOT TURN TO LEFT FINISH

Begin in OPEN CPP with weight on RF (Woman LF), facing in any direction, having danced THE CLOSE BASIC finished in OPEN CPP.

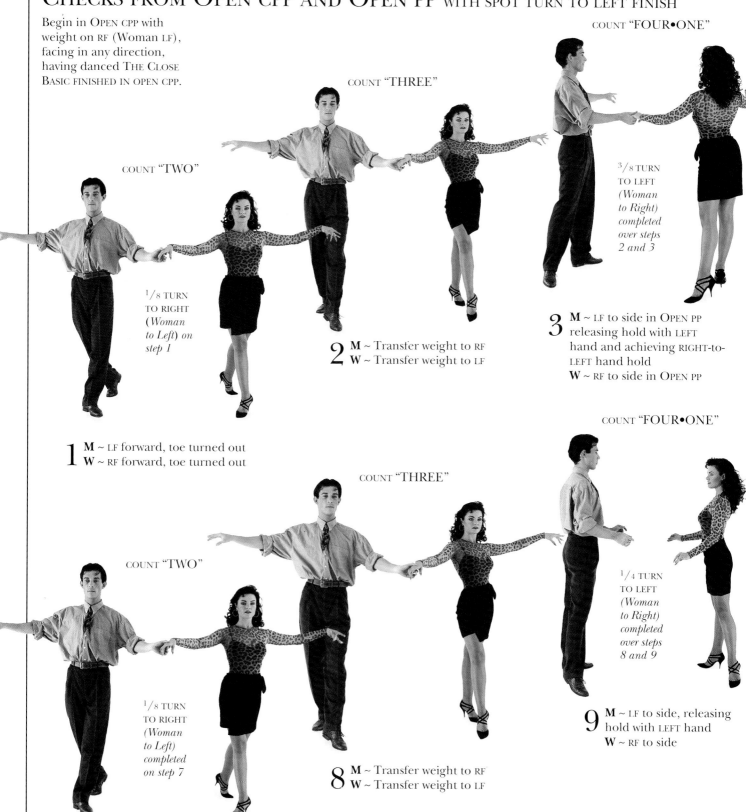

COUNT "FOUR•ONE"

COUNT "THREE"

COUNT "TWO"

1 **M** ~ LF forward, toe turned out
W ~ RF forward, toe turned out

1/8 TURN TO RIGHT (Woman to Left) on step 1

2 **M** ~ Transfer weight to RF
W ~ Transfer weight to LF

3/8 TURN TO LEFT (Woman to Right) completed over steps 2 and 3

3 **M** ~ LF to side in OPEN PP releasing hold with LEFT hand and achieving RIGHT-to-LEFT hand hold
W ~ RF to side in OPEN PP

COUNT "FOUR•ONE"

COUNT "THREE"

COUNT "TWO"

7 **M** ~ LF forward, toe turned out
W ~ RF forward, toe turned out

1/8 TURN TO RIGHT (Woman to Left) completed on step 7

8 **M** ~ Transfer weight to RF
W ~ Transfer weight to LF

1/4 TURN TO LEFT (Woman to Right) completed over steps 8 and 9

9 **M** ~ LF to side, releasing hold with LEFT hand
W ~ RF to side

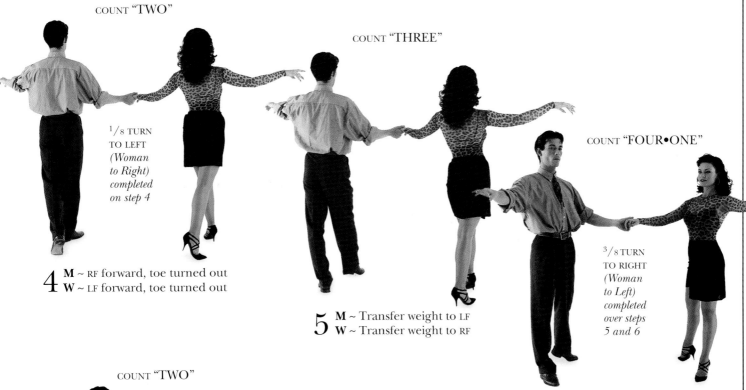

COUNT "TWO"

1/8 TURN
TO LEFT
(Woman
to Right)
completed
on step 4

4 **M** ~ RF forward, toe turned out
W ~ LF forward, toe turned out

COUNT "THREE"

5 **M** ~ Transfer weight to LF
W ~ Transfer weight to RF

COUNT "FOUR•ONE"

3/8 TURN
TO RIGHT
(Woman
to Left)
completed
over steps
5 and 6

6 **M** ~ RF to side in OPEN CPP, releasing hold with RIGHT hand, and achieving LEFT-TO-RIGHT hand hold
W ~ LF to side, in OPEN CPP

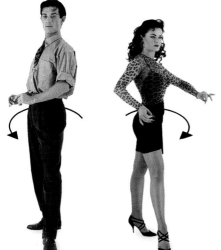

COUNT "TWO"

10 **M** ~ RF forward across LF turning strongly to LEFT to finish RF back
W ~ LF forward across RF turning strongly to RIGHT to finish LF back

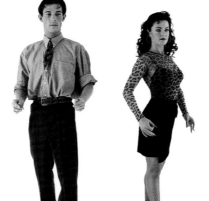

COUNT "THREE"

11 **M** ~ Transfer weight to LF
W ~ Transfer weight to RF

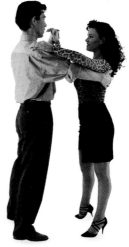

COUNT "FOUR•ONE"

ONE TURN
TO LEFT
(Woman
to Right)
completed
over steps
10, 11, 12

12 **M** ~ RF to side, achieving, CLOSE HOLD *
W ~ LF to side, achieving CLOSE HOLD *

* Continue with THE SIDE CHASSÉS AND CUCARACHAS

THE SIDE CHASSÉS AND CUCARACHAS

Begin in CLOSE HOLD, with weight on RF (Woman LF); face any direction having danced CHECKS FROM OPEN CPP and OPEN PP WITH SPOT TURN TO LEFT FINISH

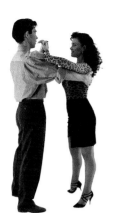

Start Position
Weight on RF
(Woman LF)

COUNT "TWO"

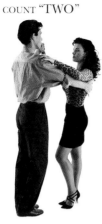

1 **M** ~ LF closed to RF
W ~ RF closed to LF

COUNT "THREE"

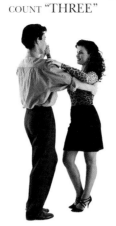

2 **M** ~ Transfer weight to RF
W ~ Transfer weight to LF

COUNT "FOUR•ONE"

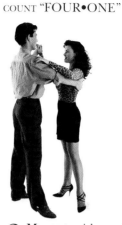

3 **M** ~ LF to side
W ~ RF to side

COUNT "TWO"

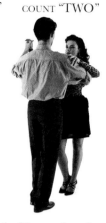

4 **M** ~ RF closed to LF
W ~ LF closed to RF

COUNT "THREE"

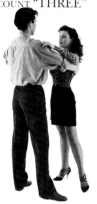

5 **M** ~ LF to side
W ~ RF to side

COUNT "FOUR•ONE"

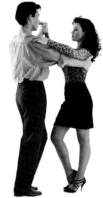

6 **M** ~ RF closed to LF
W ~ LF closed to RF

COUNT "TWO"

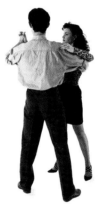

7 **M** ~ LF to side with part weight
W ~ RF to side with part weight

COUNT "THREE"

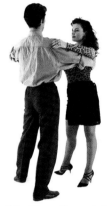

8 **M** ~ Transfer weight to RF
W ~ Transfer weight to LF

COUNT "FOUR•ONE"

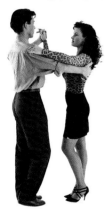

9 **M** ~ LF closed to RF
W ~ RF closed to LF

COUNT "TWO"

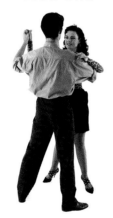

10 **M** ~ RF to side with part weight
W ~ LF to side with part weight

COUNT "THREE"

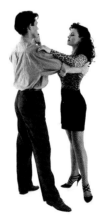

11 **M** ~ Transfer weight to LF
W ~ Transfer weight to RF

COUNT "FOUR•ONE"

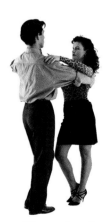

12 **M** ~ RF closed to LF *
W ~ LF closed to RF *

* Continue with THE CLOSE BASIC

GLOSSARY

AD LIB
From the Latin, *ad libitum*, meaning in accordance with one's wishes or without limit or restraint. Used here it should be read "as often as you'd like."

AMALGAMATION
Two or more figures danced one following the other. A number of different amalgamations joined together is called a *routine*.

CHASSÉ
A group of three steps, taken in any direction, during which the second step is closed or partially closed to the first step.

COUNT
Dance terminology for the time to be allocated to each step taken when dancing to music. For example, to four-in-the-bar music, the count "SLOW" denotes a step requiring two beats of music and the count "QUICK" a step that requires one beat.

COUNTER PROMENADE POSITION (CPP)
The couple assume a Vee-shape, the man's left hip being in close proximity to the woman's right hip. The man's left arm (woman's right) is raised in a soft curve just above head level.

CUCARACHA
A group of three steps taken, Side – Replace – Close. The first step is taken with part-weight in any direction. See The RUMBA, page 74, steps 7 to 12 for two examples.

FACING DIAGONALLY TO CENTRE
A position anywhere along the LOD, but having turned through an angle of 45 degrees to the left to face diagonally to an imaginary line drawn down the centre of the dance floor at that position.

FACING DIAGONALLY TO WALL
A position anywhere along the LOD, but having turned through an angle of 45 degrees to the right to face diagonally to the wall of the room at that position.

LINE OF DANCE (LOD)
This is an imaginary line around the dance floor, indicating an anticlockwise direction. A rectangular ballroom will have four lines of dance, one for each side of the room.

LOCK STEP
A group of three steps, taken forward or backward, during which the second step is crossed behind the first step, when moving forward, and is crossed in front of the first step when moving backward.

NEW LINE OF DANCE
Having negotiated a corner of the dance floor, the dancer is now ready to use the new LOD.

OPEN COUNTER PROMENADE POSITION (OPEN CPP)
Similar to COUNTER PROMENADE POSITION, but the couple have moved apart so that the man's left hip and the woman's right hip are now approximately 55 cm (22in) apart, with the man holding the woman's right hand in his left hand at about waist level.

OPEN PROMENADE POSITION (OPEN PP)
Similar to PROMENADE POSITION, but the couple have moved apart so that the man's right hip and the woman's left hip are now approximately 55 cm (22in) apart, with the man holding the woman's left hand in his right hand at about waist level.

PIVOT
A turning movement during which the dancer swivels on the ball of one of his (or her) feet while the other, weightless, foot is kept in front or behind.

PROMENADE POSITION (PP)
The couple assume a Vee-shape, the man's right hip being in close proximity to the woman's left hip. The man's left hand (woman's right) is lowered to just below shoulder level.

PREPARATORY STEP
Due to the rhythmic patterns used in Cha Cha Cha and Rumba music it is necessary to take an extra step when starting to dance these dances to music. See appropriate dance sheets for details.

FIGURES, AMALGAMATIONS, AND ROUTINES

Dancing involves moving the feet and/or body in unison with the rhythm of the music being played. Depend-ing upon the number of different movements the dancer uses to interpret the rhythm, a dance can be very simple or extremely complex. The simplest dance can be composed just of changes of weight from one foot to the other with little or no progression, but such a dance would soon become very boring. To make a dance interesting, it is necessary to include a variety of figures.

The figures that form the foundations of each dance, in dance speak, are known as basic figures. You have been learning some of these in the preceding chapters. When basic figures are danced in their correct order, they form an amalgamation. If you know only one amalgamation, it is perfectly acceptable to dance this over and over until the music stops, but as you improve your knowledge and ability, your vocabulary of figures will increase and you will be able to dance many other amalgamations.

When you join together a number of different amalgamations, this is called a routine. An accomplished male dancer should be able to introduce many varied amalgamations to produce an interesting and effective dance while making sure that they are well within the abilities of his partner, even if the couple have never danced together before.

THE BALLROOM DANCE PACK has been designed to enable beginners to take successfully to the dance floor with ease and ability and, just like millions worldwide, to gain pleasure in doing so. In order to allow you to do this in the shortest possible time, I have kept the number of figures to an absolute minimum. Different amalgamations, however, still can be created from this limited number of figures. By dancing the figures, one after the other in the order set out in the book, you have already created an amalgamation. Below, I have listed some others for each dance. They are of increasing complexity, so as your prowess grows, work your way through them. Have fun.

THE WALTZ

1. Begin in CLOSE HOLD with weight on LF (Woman RF), facing the LOD. Dance the SOLO EXERCISE with your partner and repeat *ad lib*.

2. Begin in CLOSE HOLD, with weight on LF (Woman RF), facing diagonally to wall. Dance THE QUARTER TURNS. Repeat *ad lib*. When approaching each corner of the floor turn a little more to the left on steps 7, 8, 9 and 10, 11, 12 to face diagonally to wall of the new LOD.

3. Begin in CLOSE HOLD with weight on LF (Woman RF), facing diagonally to wall. Dance THE QUARTER TURNS, THE NATURAL TURN, THE FORWARD CHANGE (RLR), THE REVERSE TURN, and THE FORWARD CHANGE (LRL). Repeat *ad lib*. When approaching each corner of the floor, dance THE NATURAL TURN to turn the corner and to finish facing diagonally to wall of the new LOD. Repeat the complete amalgamation starting with The QUARTER TURNS.

THE QUICKSTEP

1. Begin in CLOSE HOLD, with weight on LF (Woman RF), facing diagonally to wall. Dance THE QUARTER TURNS. Repeat *ad lib*. When approaching each corner of the floor, turn to LEFT on steps 5, 6, 7, 8 to face diagonally to wall of the new LOD.

2. Repeat amalgamation 1, but dance THE NATURAL PIVOT TURN when approaching each corner of the floor to finish facing diagonally to wall of the new LOD.

3. Begin in CLOSE HOLD, weight on LF (Woman RF). Dance steps 1 to 4 of THE QUARTER TURNS, then THE PROMENADE CHASSÉ, and repeat *ad lib*. When approaching each corner of the floor, follow THE PROMENADE CHASSÉ with THE NATURAL PIVOT TURN, begun by stepping forward outside your partner on her right side on step 1. Repeat *ad lib*.

4. Repeat amalgamation 3, but dance THE LOCK STEP immediately following THE PROMENADE CHASSÉ.

THE TANGO

1. Begin in CLOSE HOLD, weight on RF (Woman LF), facing diagonally to wall. Dance THE WALKS AND PROGRESSIVE SIDE STEP. Repeat *ad lib*. (This amalgamation moves in a circle and does not progress around the room, so position yourself away from the edges of the dance floor before you begin.)

2. Begin in CLOSE HOLD, weight on RF (Woman LF), facing diagonally to wall. Dance THE WALKS AND PROGRESSIVE SIDE

STEP. Repeat a WALK – LF, and a WALK – RF (Woman – RF,LF), to finish facing diagonally to centre; continue with THE REVERSE TURN. Repeat *ad lib.*

3. Begin in CLOSE HOLD, weight on RF (Woman LF), facing diagonally to wall. Dance a WALK – LF, and a WALK – RF (Woman – RF,LF); continue with THE PROGRESSIVE LINK AND CLOSED PROMENADE. Continue with amalgamation 2.

4. Repeat amalgamation 3 up to the finish of THE CLOSED PROMENADE; continue with a WALK – LF (Woman – RF), followed by NATURAL ROCK TURN. Repeat twice.

THE CHA CHA CHA

Begin in CLOSE HOLD, weight on LF (Woman RF). On the first beat of a bar of music, take a step to the side and slightly forward with RF. Then dance the following amalgamations:

1. THE CLOSE BASIC WITH UNDER ARM TURN TO RIGHT. Repeat *ad lib.*

2. Dance amalgamation 1 followed by THE CLOSE BASIC TO OPEN CPP, CHECKS FROM OPEN CPP and OPEN PP WITH SPOT TURN TO LEFT FINISH. Repeat *ad lib.*

THE SAMBA

1. Begin in CLOSE HOLD, weight on LF (Woman RF), facing the LOD. Dance THE NATURAL BASIC (twice) and THE PROGRESSIVE BASIC (twice). Repeat *ad lib.*

2. Begin in CLOSE HOLD, weight on RF (Woman LF), facing wall. Dance WHISK TO LEFT and WHISK TO RIGHT (twice), UNDER ARM TURN TO RIGHT, WHISK TO RIGHT, WHISK TO LEFT, and UNDER ARM TURN TO LEFT. Repeat *ad lib.*

3. Dance amalgamation 2 followed by WHISK TO LEFT, WHISK TO RIGHT turned to PP, SAMBA WALK (LRL) in PP and SAMBA WALK (RLR) in PP. Repeat SAMBA WALK (LRL) in PP and SAMBA WALK (RLR) in PP. Continue by dancing WHISK TO LEFT turned to CLOSE HOLD. Repeat *ad lib.*

THE RUMBA

Begin in CLOSE HOLD, weight on LF (Woman RF). On the fourth beat of a bar of music, take a step to the side and slightly forward on the RF. Then dance the following amalgamations:

1. Dance THE CLOSE BASIC WITH UNDER ARM TURN TO RIGHT. Repeat *ad lib.*

2. Dance amalgamation 1, followed by THE CLOSE BASIC FINISHED IN OPEN CPP, CHECKS FROM OPEN CPP and OPEN PP WITH SPOT TURN TO LEFT FINISH. Repeat *ad lib.*

3. Dance amalgamation 2 followed by THE CLOSE BASIC WITH UNDER ARM TURN TO RIGHT, and THE SIDE CHASSÉS AND CUCARACHAS. Continue with amalgamation 1, 2, or 3.

LEADING AND FOLLOWING

Ballroom dancing is a form of together-dancing – either the couple's bodies are in contact or the partners hold hands. The man determines the figures to be danced and their order. It is his role to control and lead his partner throughout each dance; the woman's response is to follow the man's lead.

Normally, the woman is not aware in advance of the figures her partner will use while dancing with her, so the man must be able to communicate his intentions to his partner. He does so through leading.

The arts of leading and following the many compli-cated movements used by top-class dancers take years to master. But social dancers, too, need to understand and learn the fundamental principles right from the beginning. The rewards are enormous. You will not only be able to dance with comfort and ease, but there is delight in moving in perfect harmony with the music. Although time and effort are required to ensure that brain, body, and emotions are co-ordinated, it is certainly worth making the effort.

To become an accomplished male social dancer requires considerable skill. After inviting a woman to dance, the man must start by using the simplest of figures – figures that require a minimum of dancing ability from the woman. Then, gradually, the man should introduce more figures that he is really confident that he can lead, so allowing his partner to have a comfortable, unstressful, enjoyable dance.

When in doubt, keep it simple; your partner will appreciate your thoughtfulness and expertise.

WHAT SHALL I WEAR?

Social dancing is the avocation of millions of people in many different countries throughout the world. These dedicated people dance anywhere suitable music is played and there is sufficient space. The space required can be a night-club floor, just big enough to swing a cat, or an enormous ballroom floor as large as a football field. It could be in the open air under a canopy of brilliant stars, where casually dressed people may congregate after a day on the beach, or it could be in a palace on a grand State occasion, crowded with men in their white ties and well-cut tail suits with their partners dressed in beautiful evening gowns with diamond-studded ornamentation adorning their necks and fingers.

Competition dancers spend a great deal of time, effort, and money on clothes that will complement their dance routines; the female dancers shown in THE BALLROOM DANCE PACK, wear a different gown or dress for each dance. And while tails are suitable for all Modern dances, our male Latin dancer sports a new outfit for each of his. For social dancers, however, the answer to the question "What shall I wear?" when going dancing, is not dictated so much by the dancing, but by the occasion and venue where the dancing is to take place. It's your night out; be comfortable and enjoy it.

FOR WOMEN ONLY

Personal choice will determine colour and type but it is important to bear in mind that the design and style of dress you choose could affect your performance on the dance floor. A few pointers, therefore, may help to ensure a successful evening.

Usually, you will be dancing a mixture of Modern and Latin dances, so you must be careful to choose a style of dress that gives you sufficient freedom of leg action, while dancing the Modern dances. Also, the same dress must be suitable for the Latin dances. Latin dances are more static and the body actions often used to express the rhythm include some figures that require the woman to make fairly fast turns; these often make the skirt of the dress rise. During the Latin dances you will be moving your arms and shoulders quite freely, so do not wear a dress with a strapless top that is held in place with a zip unless you are sure it will not move around – or worse, part company with your body while you are on the dance floor.

Finally, do not wear a hairstyle that could collapse around your ears after a few fast turns, and avoid earrings that could part company with your earlobes after a sharp turn of your head.

DANCE SHOES AND FLOORS

Whether you are a beginner or an advanced dancer, there is one item of your dress that must be correct to ensure a pleasant and safe evening's dancing. This is your footwear.

If you are to dance on a beach, in a car park, or in a barn, almost any type of shoe will suffice, but if you are to dance on smooth wood or a marble floor take care! It is amazing how people, who are responsible for laying floors intended to be suitable for dancing, do not understand what is the best floor surface for any form of ballroom dancing, nor do those, who prepare these floors for a night's dancing, know how it should be prepared. Many people believe that ballroom dancers require a smooth, slippery surface but this is complete nonsense. Yes, of course, dancers require a smooth surface on which to dance, but not a hard floor polished to a mirror finish.

The perfect dancing floor is one consisting of Canadian Maple or a similar wood that is sprung when laid to give a soft feel. The surface should be prepared to provide an acceptable degree of friction between the sole of the dancer's shoe and the floor surface. Dancers need some friction from the floor to create movement; it is impossible to dance on a sheet of ice. So please be careful. Never dance on a floor with a slippery surface when wearing new shoes – shoes with a smooth shiny leather sole. At best, you will not enjoy your evening's dancing; at worst, you could have a nasty fall. New shoes need to be prepared beforehand.

PREPARING NEW DANCE SHOES

There are two ways of ensuring new shoes' suitability for the dance floor. The first way to give new shoes some grip, is to rough up their smooth leather soles with a file or coarse sandpaper. The second, and by far the best way, is the method used by all professional ballroom dancers: first rough up the smooth leather soles as explained above; then cover each sole completely with a piece of split-chrome leather that has been previously cut to a size slightly larger than the sole. Stick one of these pieces on to each sole using a rubber-based adhesive. Finally, trim to exactly the size of the sole of each shoe. Men should also cover the heel of each shoe.

Split-chrome leather and suitable adhesives can be obtained from most shoe repairers. And, if you are not a do-it-yourself person, I am sure you can find a shoe repairer who will do the job for you. Alternatively, you can purchase shoes already fitted with split-chrome leather soles.

Remember, the only physical contact you have with the world when you are dancing is through the soles (and heels) of your shoes; make sure this is a safe contact.

Since the type of shoe worn while dancing can affect the performance of all dancers, from beginners to champions, the following information gives some guidance on shoes that are most suitable for Modern and Latin styles of ballroom dancing.

SHOES FOR MEN

Modern ballroom dance shoes for men can be of plain leather, patent, or a mixture of leather and suede. Some shoes are perforated for ventilation, particularly those worn for practice sessions. Heels are normally 2.5cm (1 in) high.

Latin shoes for men are often made of imitation suede, which is long lasting, or of very soft calf. The heels are normally as for Modern shoes though some men prefer the higher (4cm/1½ in) Cuban heel.

When choosing dancing shoes, the most important criterion is that they must be comfortable on the foot – preferably rather a snug fit, not loose. The design should be of the lace-up variety and not slip-on; the sole should be thinner and more flexible than that of a normal walking shoe.

For more dressy occasions, if you choose to wear shoes with high-gloss material uppers, be aware that there is a dangerous tendency for some types of this material to stick when the feet are closed or when one foot is brushed past the other. In all other matters, such as choice of style and design and height of heels, personal choice can be your guide.

SHOES FOR WOMEN

Top-class lady exponents of the two dancing styles, Modern and Latin, use a different type of shoe for each.

The most suitable shoe for Modern dances is a Court shoe (one without an ankle strap) with a 5–6.25cm (2–2½ in) heel. Usually, these shoes are made of white satin which can be dyed to match the colour of the dress to be worn, but plain coloured or metallic leathers are also available.

A sandal-type shoe with a 6.25–7.5cm (2½–3 in) slimmer heel and an ankle strap is the preferred style for Latin dancing; the open toes facilitate many of the movements. Silver- or gold-coloured leather styles are popular, but shoes can also be of white satin, dyed to suit the dress to be worn.

Both types of shoe are often sold with suede soles to add grip and prevent you slipping.

Remember, whatever type of shoe you choose for your ballroom dancing, it must be flexible, fit the foot snugly and be comfortable to wear.

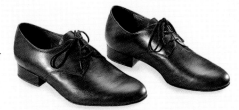

Shoe may have perforations for ventilation

Plain leather Modern shoes

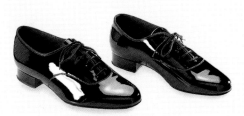

Patent leather Modern shoes

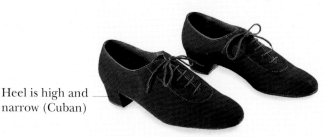

Heel is high and narrow (Cuban)

Suede Latin shoes

Elasticated front will grip foot

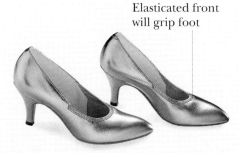

Leather Court Modern shoes

T-bar construction relieves pressure on ankle

Open toes permit movement

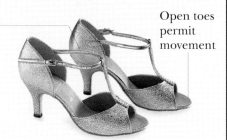

Fabric (glitter effect) Latin sandals

ACKNOWLEDGEMENTS

Carroll & Brown Limited were fortunate to be able to work with Walter Laird, a true professional and champion who provided the words, the dancers, the expertise, and great good humour. We are also grateful for the invaluable assistance Julie Laird provided with the production of THE BALLROOM DANCE PACK.

The professional dancers who interpreted the dance steps made the book come alive, and we thank them for their efforts in achieving this. In the Modern section, Kate Fisher and Paul Holmes danced The WALTZ, The QUICKSTEP, and The TANGO. In the Latin section, Vibeke Toft and Allan Tornsberg performed The CHA CHA CHA, The SAMBA, and The RUMBA. We also used photographs of Tone Nyhagen and Martin Dihlmann performing the Latin dances.

Supadance Shoes provided the footwear for page 79, and Patricia Shine did the original research.

Chris Craker wrote and produced some marvellous music for the compact disc, which was enthusiastically performed by The London Ballroom Dance Band.

Chloe Alexander of Dorling Kindersley Ltd. created an enticing jacket.

Editorial Amy Carroll
Madeline Weston

Design Denise Brown
Hans Verkroost
Alan Watt

Typesetting
Debbie Lelliott
DTP

Production Lorraine Baird
Wendy Rogers
Amanda Mackie

Photography David Murray

Artwork André-Scott Bamforth
Aziz Khan